W9-AYO-856

Date: 6/1/20

WHAT SCIENCE TELLS US ABOUT AUTISM SPECTRUM DISORDER

Also Available

WHAT SCIENCE TELLS US ABOUT AUTISM SPECTRUM DISORDER

Making the Right Choices for Your Child

Raphael A. Bernier, PhD
Geraldine Dawson, PhD
Joel T. Nigg, PhD

THE GUILFORD PRESS
NEW YORK   LONDON

Copyright © 2020 The Guilford Press
A Division of Guilford Publications, Inc.
370 Seventh Avenue, Suite 1200, New York, NY 10001
www.guilford.com

Printed in the United States of America

This book is printed on acid-free paper.

Last digit is print number: 9   8   7   6   5   4   3   2   1

Library of Congress Cataloging-in-Publication Data is available from the publisher.

ISBN 978-1-4625-3607-8 (paperback)— ISBN 978-1-4625-4137-9 (hardcover)

CONTENTS

INTRODUCTION

Autism spectrum disorder is among the most visible and well-known conditions affecting brain development. Few people cannot name some connection to or story about an individual with autism. Reports in the news about scientific breakthroughs and human interest stories chronicling the lives of families affected by autism are commonplace. If you do a simple Internet search for "autism," you'll find about 144 million results in about half a second. Put simply, there is a lot of information—and perhaps also a lot of noise—out there about autism spectrum disorder, or ASD for short, and there are many misconceptions and differing reports regarding the causes, treatments, and even what ASD is.

There are plenty of reasons for this, including highly effective advocacy by stakeholders in the community. However, one huge reason for this tidal wave of information and misinformation is that our awareness and scientific understanding of ASD are changing and advancing at a blazing speed. These rapid advances mean practical, tangible, impactful opportunities that you can take advantage of to make a big difference to your child's health, happiness, and well-being, and that of your family.

In this book we've sifted through the volume of information and misinformation to give you a clear understanding of what science tells us about ASD—and how it can be applied to help your child. We outline the key recent advances in neuroscience and genetics, highlighting those that have real-world, practical implications for your child. And, because a diagnosis of autism impacts the family in addition to the child, changes in your child with autism will reverberate in your family. We will delve into what science has taught us about sleep, exercise, diet, and the gastro-intestinal system in ASD and flag what you can do with this information to start making changes today. We will provide no-nonsense advice about how to put together a treatment package that works for you and your family specifically—because no one approach will work for all families. And we will critically examine and dissect the misconceptions and myths that continue to haunt parents, clinicians, and the media today, so that you can rest assured that you're making the right choices for your child and your family.

This book will help you:

- Learn what recent research has revealed about autism and how to distinguish scientific evidence from unfounded or exaggerated claims

- Get a handle on where your child falls on the autism spectrum and how that can guide your choices of interventions

- Learn how to find the most appropriate treatment for your child

- Separate fact from fiction about what causes ASD

- See how lifestyle changes around sleep, nutrition, and exercise can impact your child with autism and identify practical tips to make those lifestyle changes

- Understand the steps you can take as your child transitions into adolescence and into adulthood

- Keep up with new science and future research directions

HOW TO USE THIS BOOK

The first four chapters of this book share the new science of ASD—what we know about the causes, how ASD develops, and how the brain works differently in ASD. These chapters provide the foundation for the rest of the book, so we propose that everyone read Chapters 1–4. Built on this foundation, you'll find six chapters about what the latest research findings tell us that you can do to help your child achieve the best possible quality of life. These chapters offer the details on what we know about how modifications to the environment and lifestyle can change how your child's brain grows and how your child's behaviors take shape. We encourage you to review the table of contents and then read Chapters 5–10 in whatever order best fits your interests. Each chapter translates the findings from the state-of-the-art science in ASD on topics such as sleep, exercise, diet, and technology into practical strategies for you to apply to your family and your child's daily life toward a happier and healthier life for everyone. For most children with ASD who are struggling with social communication and interaction, some form of professional help will be an important element in treatment. In Chapter 5 you'll find the latest science on professionally guided interventions and how to assemble your treatment team. In Chapters 6–8 we'll bring our new understanding of ASD to sleep, exercise, diet, gastrointestinal troubles, and technology. In Chapters 9 and 10 we explain what research shows about what works best in life for adolescents and, looking ahead, adults with ASD. In Chapter 11 we'll bring all of this new understanding together so that you can decide on a course of action as your child develops through adolescence and early adulthood. Here you'll read a variety of stories that illustrate how the science can be applied to diverse children, teens, and adults. These stories, and others throughout the book, are based on composites of real people we have known and worked with and represent common situations and challenges along the spectrum.

All of the information and advice you'll find in this book reflects two overarching themes that the latest science has uncovered. First, ASD is not a singular condition, a realization that has implications for how we provide supports. Second, there are specific supports that we can put in place now that can result in very positive outcomes for many children. Autism can no longer be viewed as a "life sentence."

ASD Takes Different Shapes in Different Individuals

Although "autism" is a single word and a single diagnostic label, autism is not a singular thing. There is a saying in the world of autism that if you've met one child with autism, you've met one child with autism. Although the diagnostic criteria are clear enough, a vast spectrum of different challenges and abilities fits within those criteria. For example, each child with ASD has social deficits in some form, but they look very different from child to child. For one child those social deficits may mean the child doesn't share or show others his latest Lego construction or the school assignment he just completed. For another it may mean the child sticks to a conversational topic despite seemingly clear messages that the conversation is definitely over. In the same vein, similar patterns of inflexible thinking may be reflected in one child's having a meltdown when taken home from school by a different route than usual; for another it may appear in lined-up toys or impeccably arranged stuffed animals that cannot be moved from their spot. Similarly, while many people with autism have areas of exceptional skill, the nature of those skills varies widely—from art to math to music.

How do we get such wondrous variety within a supposedly single medical condition? Well, to start, the causes of autism are more complex than once thought. As recently as a decade ago many scientists guessed that only a handful of genes would be involved. There is in fact no single unitary cause of autism. The causes are usually complex, and they are many. While genetics plays a significant role in autism, we now estimate that at least a thousand genes and genetic events play a role in the development of autism. While many of these genes interact and are related, they are still distinct. These genes provide the code for proteins that perform functions as diverse as guiding how brain cells connect to how genes turn on and off in the cell nuclei to how brain cells allow the passage of molecules across their membranes. Each of these distinct processes brings different effects on the brain that intersect in a wide variety of ways. Things get even more complicated by the fact that these combined genetic effects interact with a child's developmental history, learning, and personality. The result is a nearly infinite number of different behaviors that we might see in children with the same syndrome.

As just implied, it's crucial to remember that genes don't act alone; they interact with other genes, and, contrary to some misconceptions, they always interact with their environment. And by environment, we're not referring to mountains or rain. Rather, in the case of autism, the relevant environment begins with maternal and paternal experiences even before conception, continuing through pregnancy and into early life and then through development. It includes factors as diverse as teratogens (elements that cause malformation) during prenatal development, lack of oxygen perinatally, and others that we'll review.

The recognition that autism is not a singular thing is critical to understanding the need to individualize your plans for your child with ASD. A single treatment approach will not be effective for every child. When you know that autism has many different causes and follows many different courses, you and your child's support team can focus on identifying the appropriate interventions for your particular child at any given time.

THERE ARE MANY WAYS TO IMPROVE THE OUTCOME FOR YOUR CHILD

A generation ago, a diagnosis of autism was seen as a life sentence. There were few options, scant resources, limited information, and little hope for children and families. The story is very different today. Recent research has demonstrated how many different paths and steps are available to help your child. And one of the critical messages is that you, as the caregiver, can be the most powerful ingredient in creating the necessary opportunities for growth and change for your child.

Today we have a much better understanding of what the essence of the autism spectrum is. That understanding has improved our ability to identify autism earlier and get children on the appropriate developmental path when the brain is most plastic (meaning adaptable) and responsive to intervention. Importantly, today's interventions can—at least for some children—effectively address the core challenges of autism. We also know what associated challenges to keep our eyes peeled for and have approaches to address many of those challenges. All of this means improved quality of life for your child and your family.

The impact of this new science cannot be underestimated. *While 50 years ago autism was almost always a permanently disabling condition, nowadays a growing proportion of children with ASD, as they get older, and with the support of the family and their community, no longer meet the diagnostic criteria for autism.* For those who do remain on the spectrum, proper support can lead to a fulfilling and productive life. In fact, many adults on the ASD spectrum now take pride in their unique talents and perspectives, realizing that diversity contributes to the success of all of humankind. Thus, our aim here is not to change who your child is but to help you maximize your child's capabilities and opportunities to choose freely and develop into the person he wants to be.

As we'll describe, those important steps that you can take include assembling your treatment package from an informed perspective guided by best practices, what the science tells us, and simple guidelines that help you evaluate the appropriateness of a given treatment for your child and family. Arming yourself with knowledge about the essential components of an evaluation and basic educational rights provides you with the support to ensure your child is at the center of the treatment program. Beyond general knowledge, knowledge about the situational drivers of your child's specific behaviors is critical. The best way to gain that knowledge is to follow the clues the way a detective might. As we'll discuss throughout this book, there are ways to examine your child's behavior systematically so you can identify the cause of the behavior. And by understanding the cause, you or your team can better intervene and incorporate that understanding into the treatment package.

Lifestyle has proven more beneficial, when harnessed properly, than previously thought. The most recent scientific research also shows that we cannot underestimate the influence of sleep and exercise on your child's behavior and learning. By adopting key strategies for ensuring healthy sleep and exercise patterns as we describe in Chapter 6, you can prep your child and her brain to be healthy and optimally responsive to learning about the social world and ready to replace challenging behaviors with new, adaptive strategies. Similarly, as we'll describe in Chapter 7, diet and nutrition must be considered, especially given the increased rates of gastrointestinal problems seen in many children with ASD and recent breakthroughs in understanding how the gut and brain talk to one another. Commonsense approaches to ensuring that your child's diet is nutritionally appropriate and paths to take to address the GI problems common in the autism community are available.

Advances in the application of technology in ASD are widely discussed today, but we will advise a balance between the promise of technology and appropriate caution about the perils it holds. We review steps you can take to support your child with technology while avoiding the pitfalls.

And finally, scientific advances have provided avenues to support your child as he grows into adolescence and matures into adulthood. This transition can be as intimidating as your child's first day in kindergarten; fortunately, you can take some clearly defined steps to weather this period. These include simple steps to emphasize good hygiene and practical aspects of daily living and helping to support your child's involvement in the community. They also include concrete steps in the adolescent years around setting in place guardianship or financial supports, if appropriate for your family, that will ease the transition period and reduce the stress of that stage of life. All of the concrete steps that we'll discuss in this book are based on our integration of the incredible new advances in the science of autism.

WHAT DOES THE FUTURE HOLD FOR AUTISM?

We can't foresee the future with perfect clarity, of course, but we can consider the trends in scientific advances made in the past quarter century and make well-informed guesses that we and you can act on. In psychology there is a truism that the best predictor of future behavior is past behavior, and we can extend that to psychological and medical science. The gains we've made in our understanding of autism are astounding compared to what was once believed possible. Each day we gain more insights into the specific causes of autism, build confidence in our empirically supported treatments, and develop new ways to increase access and opportunities for learning for families affected by autism. Just 10 years ago we did not even know which genes were related to autism. We now have a confirmed list of over 200 specific genes that are linked to it (in Chapter 3, we'll delve into this subject in detail). Just 10 years ago behaviorally based treatments were not reimbursed by insurance companies, making the only scientifically validated treatment for autism out of financial reach for most families (in Chapter 5, we'll discuss interventions). And, just 10 years ago we had no idea what was happening in the brain for individuals with autism, and now we understand the brain circuitry and relevant changes that contribute to the challenges (and strengths) that individuals with autism show (we'll discuss the brain in Chapter 4). That trajectory of advances will undoubtedly continue at the same rapid rate. Throughout this book we'll highlight the latest research and hint at what the next steps are so that you stay on the cutting edge of what the science of autism has to offer.

We hope that you take away from this book a hopeful, yet well-grounded understanding of how ASD develops and how it can change over time. With this fresh look at the science, we hope you are freed from any remaining self-blame and hopelessness and instead are empowered and prepared to take the steps that you can to create the best possible life for your child and family.

1

A New Understanding
of Autism Spectrum Disorder

Autism was initially described in the 1940s as a single disorder of child-hood. The hallmark symptoms described at that time are likely famil-iar to you: the children seen then, like children today with autism, had substantial difficulty with social interactions and communication and a restricted range of interests and behaviors. These still-classic features are seen in behaviors such as reduced eye contact, limited facial expressions, and unusual ways of interacting with other people. You may have noticed that along with unusually narrow and often intense interests, many chil-dren with autism are also highly sensitive to certain touches, textures, sounds, or sights—and prefer the same routine every day.

While these features are essentially how we still describe autism today, we have a more nuanced understanding of the life path for those with autism. Symptoms are rarely noticeable during the first 6 months of life and typically emerge at around 8–12 months. However, for about a third of children who will develop autism, development is apparently nor-mal until toddlerhood, followed by a loss of skills at that time. Regard-less of the developmental timing, autism severity varies widely—some individuals live and work independently; others cannot. Some develop adequate language skills; some never develop language. For most, the challenges are lifelong, but every child makes progress and acquires skills, although at widely varying rates. In other words, it is certain that not every single thing we say about autism will apply to your child.

In fact, while scientists treated autism as a single condition for decades, it no longer makes sense to do so. Kids with autism differ so much from each other that it's vital to take the general principles we'll cover and then tailor them to your individual child. You have no doubt already begun that process; we'll make more suggestions as we go. For now, it's important to realize that science agrees with many parents' intuition that there are many different kinds of autism.

These differences can be vast. Parents whose child cannot talk or do any math will wonder how their child can have the same condition as a child who can do algebra or explain the periodic table of elements.

Likewise, while the causes are only partially understood, we are confident now that there is more than one cause of autism. In fact, the latest scientific view is that ASD is a collection of several related conditions, with identifiable and partially shared characteristics. This new understanding has paved the way for major gains in understanding the causes—and new hope for effective treatments for children with ASD.

Although this book explains many recent advances in our understanding of ASD, some of the most significant to the outcomes we can expect for children with the disorder—and the most important for parents to be aware of—are the following.

Autism Falls Along a Spectrum

Let's start with the idea that autism occurs along a spectrum, a concept that is now generally accepted by researchers and clinicians. Before we delve into what we mean when we use the word "spectrum," how did we get from autism as a single disorder to a spectrum?

The Evolution of the Diagnosis

Clinicians use a common system to diagnose mental health and developmental disorders. The *Diagnostic and Statistical Manual of Mental Disorders* (DSM) is the guidebook for diagnosing a wide range of conditions affecting mental health and development. Developed shortly after World War II to standardize psychiatric terminology, and now published by the American Psychiatric Association, the manual has been revised significantly over the years and now includes conditions affecting brain development and behavior in children. It is now in its fifth edition (DSM-5), which came out in 2013. Intended to guide clinicians, the DSM lists the criteria that must be met to make a valid diagnosis; other factors that should be taken into account, such as what other diagnoses should be considered; and current information about the disorder, such as its prevalence, known causes, and the physiological aspects of the disorder. The listed criteria generally include parameters for what symptoms or behaviors must be present, how long they must be present, and when they first began. But the pattern of behaviors also must cause significant impairments in social, vocational, or educational functioning. In other words, by definition, the behaviors must be causing impairments in the child's life. If they don't result in any challenges in these domains, they will not be defined as a disorder in the DSM.

Autism as an independent entity was first included as an entry in 1980 in the third edition of the DSM (DSM-III) under the label "infantile autism." In 1987 the American Psychiatric Association published a revised edition (DSM-III-R) in which the term "autistic disorder" was presented with some more formalized criteria based on new statistical analyses. In 1994, DSM-IV was published. Autistic disorder remained but was joined by associated conditions under the umbrella term "pervasive developmental disorders" (PDD). The umbrella included autistic disorder, Asperger syndrome, and PDD-not otherwise specified (these three subgroups became the future "spectrum") as well as Rett syndrome and childhood disintegrative disorder. Other associated terms, like nonverbal learning disorder, were excluded because they were not considered scientifically rigorous. Thus, for nearly two decades, from 1994 to 2013, we attempted to study and treat autism within three official subcategories: autistic disorder, Asperger syndrome, and PDD.

However, as we detail in a moment, that effort to create subtypes failed. In 2013, the new DSM-5 eliminated the subcategories, such as Asperger syndrome versus autistic disorder, and created a single autism spectrum disorder—thus broadening the autism criteria and simplifying the diagnosing clinician's task. The current criteria essentially cover what we've already mentioned—social communication and interaction challenges and narrow and/or repetitive behaviors that appear early in life and cause significant impairments.

Why was this done? While the initial years following psychiatrist Leo Kanner's identification of ASD in the 1940s were focused on describing the commonalities in ASD, over the years the broad range of challenges, strengths, and variability became apparent—culminating in the ill-fated attempt in DSM-IV to create formal subcategories. Several findings convinced the field to drop the separate diagnoses for Asperger syndrome and PDD. An important factor was that there were no treatments specific to the different subgroups. That is, there were no standardized differences in how a child diagnosed with Asperger syndrome and another child diagnosed with autistic disorder would be treated.

More crucially, it turned out that expert clinicians were not very reliable at determining which children should be assigned to which diagnostic subclassification. One decisive finding in 2012 that helped solidify the importance of conceptualizing autism as a spectrum disorder and not three distinct subgroups illustrates this. It involved the evaluation of diagnostic practices for 2,000 children across 12 university-based centers in North America where the research clinics were all conducting diagnostic evaluations for autism in the same exact way. At each site, expert clinicians at these top institutions used gold-standard diagnostic tools to assess autism and administered a standardized battery of tests to assess other features such as cognition and language. To ensure that everyone was conducting assessments in exactly the same way and following the proper DSM-IV guidelines, all the evaluations were videotaped. The final analysis showed that there were no differences in the types of children in the study—no one site saw more children with intellectual disability or more children with language impairment or irritability or motor problems or any of the other hundreds of variables—yet the clinicians arrived at radically different rates of the subclassifications. One site only diagnosed children with autistic disorder. Another site diagnosed over half of the children with Asperger syndrome. Another site didn't diagnose any children with PDD. In other words, the clinicians agreed that these children all met diagnostic criteria for the umbrella term "autism" but could not agree on the subclassification. The take-home message was that even the top diagnosticians in North America failed to consistently or effectively use the behaviorally based subclassifications. Finally, no convincing biological differences among the subtypes had been found either.

WHY IS THERE A SPECTRUM?

The autism spectrum includes these former subcategories, as well as variation in severity and profile of symptoms. Scientists believe autism occurs along a spectrum because the core features take so many different shapes, and we now have evidence that the core deficits in the disorder develop along many different causal pathways involving different biological systems as well as different genetic and environmental inputs. To increase our understanding of the science behind autism, therefore, we now study the entire spectrum, and as we'll discuss, this approach has already paid off with clearer biological findings.

By recognizing there is a broad spectrum, scientists can use brain imaging, genetics, and other cutting-edge scientific approaches to understand the variability in the spectrum. In turn, the information we gain helps us develop treatment plans that will benefit a diverse population on the spectrum and design novel interventions and ultimately be better individualized for a given child.

One way to understand the different faces of autism, or subtypes, involves genetics. Genetic information has been helpful in doing the same thing for other conditions, such as intellectual and learning disabilities. A little over a century ago, all children with intellectual disability were considered to have the same condition. We now know, however, that intellectual disability, like ASD, is a behaviorally defined disorder with many causes. It gradually became clear, for example, that some intellectual disability ran in families and some did not, suggesting there were different causes. Over time many single-gene causes of intellectual disability have been discovered, to the point where today more than 1,000 such rare conditions are known. Yet other kinds of intellectual disability do not have single-gene causes.

One well-known example of a single-gene cause is the genetic disorder called phenylketonuria, or PKU. Prior to the identification of that gene mutation, children with PKU were simply diagnosed with intellectual disability based on their symptoms. But the discovery that the gene associated with PKU is responsible for processing phenylalanine in the body ultimately led to a simple route to preventing PKU. Babies can be given a heel-stick test at birth, and when it's positive, prevention of this subtype of intellectual disability is a simple matter of omitting from the baby's diet the many foods containing phenylalanine. While the story is unlikely to end that way for ASD, the logic is similar—the biological and causal groupings will not be obvious on the surface, but much can be learned that will ultimately help kids at various points along the spectrum.

To elaborate on genetics for a moment, we've known that genetics plays a role in autism since the first twin studies in the 1970s. Since then many different genetic inputs have been identified for autism. As we'll discuss in Chapter 2, about 1,000 different genes and genomic regions are implicated in autism. Although these do not determine who will have ASD in the same way they do for some of the 1,000 kinds of intellectual disability, the findings do suggest that autism is probably best seen as a set of many related conditions and there are different pathways to developing the symptoms that we call autism. Finding out what, if anything, these gene effects have in common will be an important future goal for research. In subsequent chapters we will elaborate on what is known about both genetic and environmental influences on ASD.

Severity and Level of Impairment

Until scientists can pin down certain subtypes based on biology, genes, or environmental causes, parents and clinicians can get information about how to help each particular child by understanding where the child falls along the spectrum. Where any individual child is on the spectrum depends to a great extent on the severity of the condition as well as the child's developmental level and chronological age. Very generally speaking, if the defining features of autism are fairly severe and impairing in a child, and the child has a developmental level much lower than is typical at that chronological age (say, a developmental level of age 3 in a 12-year-old), the child is on the end of the spectrum that will necessitate lots of support and intervention. But as recent research has shown, that very support and intervention can eventually improve the child's condition and reduce how much help the child needs in daily life going forward.

We like the spectrum idea because it can help us focus on the individual profile, the specific strengths and challenges a child has. This individualized attention allows for plans that incorporate strengths a child may have, such as visual processing or rote memorization, to offset challenges in social processing or difficulties with transitions.

Aside from these autism-specific symptoms, research done in the last 20 years tells us that there is an array of other conditions often associated with autism, and these will also affect what kind of treatment and support an individual child needs. This is why it's so important for parents and clinicians to identify such factors in each child being diagnosed. It's not just the core symptoms that need to be addressed to produce a good outcome for the child but these other conditions too.

MANY OTHER CONDITIONS AFFECT CHILDREN WITH ASD

One of the most obvious ways that children with autism differ from one another is the other conditions that frequently occur alongside of autism. These include physical as well as behavioral conditions. The reason for these frequent overlaps, while they are an important potential clue to causes, is generally not well known. However, the strong overlap of these conditions has been part of the motivation for the increasing contemporary scientific view that ASD and several of the conditions listed here constitute a family of related conditions associated with specific, yet-to-be-identified alterations in early brain development and growth.

Intellectual Disability

The first of these to understand is *intellectual disability*—a term that replaces older and now stigmatizing terms like "mental retardation." It basically means that the individual's intellectual abilities are not as developed as they are for most people who are the same age, and that, furthermore, the individual's practical life skills (what your child's clinician might call "adaptive" skills) are also less developed. These include practical skills like bathing and using money without help. About a third of people who have autism spectrum disorder also have intellectual disability. Intellectual disability can range from mild (perhaps not obvious to the layperson) to severe. If your child falls into the latter group, then additional special supports will be involved in helping him. We'll come to this again in Chapter 5.

Language and Communication Disorders

Another condition that is commonly associated with autism is delayed or reduced language development. Language impairments vary and can range from a child having minimal or no spoken language, which occurs in about 15% of children with ASD, to a child who has unusual speech, such as repeating scripted words or phrases or echoing back what someone has just said (called "echolalia"), to those whose speech is not significantly impaired. Other types of atypical language use include the use of invented words (called "neologisms"), like using the word "coo-is-a-car" to refer to trees, or the use of pronoun reversals such as referring to oneself in third person or mixing up "you" for "I" when asking a question. For example, a child who asks "You want a glass of milk?" may actually mean "I want a glass of milk." Other children may have difficulties only in expressing themselves in words (called "expressive language") but be able to understand language much better (called "receptive language"). Children who have little spoken language can benefit from using technology, such as a tablet or other devices, to communicate and learn. Fortunately, with therapy, all children can learn to communicate, whether through words or other means.

ADHD

Attention-deficit/hyperactivity disorder (ADHD) is a common syndrome, also with a spectrum of severity, that describes individuals who are extremely inattentive, unable to stay focused or organized, or else are extremely overactive (as if always driven by a motor) or extremely impulsive. As many as half of children with ASD have substantial problems with inattention or hyperactivity and would also meet criteria for a diagnosis of ADHD. Just since DSM-5 in 2013, clinicians are now allowed to codiagnose and treat both disorders. For some children problems with hyperactivity and difficulties regulating behavior can exacerbate existing social challenges because over time peers can become frustrated and withdraw from a child who is impulsive and hyperactive. That further restricts the opportunities for the child with ASD to practice and learn social skills. If your child is in this group, your treating clinicians may recommend medications for ADHD (in addition to the commonly known

Ritalin [methylphenidate], a dozen other formulations are available that can be helpful). We now know, from recent studies, that children with ASD who also meet criteria for ADHD can in fact benefit from such medicines. If the primary problem here is not hyperactivity but attention, the clinician may also recommend special skills training related to attention, to help, for example, with schoolwork. The potential lifestyle and alternative treatment proposals for ADHD and ASD overlap heavily, although the data gathered on what works reveal some differentiation between these conditions too. Interested parents may find more information about ADHD in Joel Nigg's book *Getting Ahead of ADHD*.

Emotional Problems

Kids with ASD can experience emotional complications too. We live in a social world, and if you struggle to make your way through social situations, it's not hard to imagine that you would be susceptible to feeling anxious and sad. As you might predict, we often see higher rates of anxiety and mood disorders, like depression, in those with ASD— particularly in teens and adults who have more insight into their differences. Individuals with ASD who have limited language or difficulties with understanding their own emotional experiences will have trouble telling people about their feelings of anxiety or sadness. But you may be able to see it in your child's behavior, such as being overly fearful or losing interest in activities the child used to enjoy. If your child is in this group, a behavioral plan that takes into account the anxiety or mood concern can be helpful, as can methods to reduce stress and improve stress-related coping, all skills your clinician may recommend as part of your child's treatment.

Medical Issues

Medical concerns that occur more often than we would expect with ASD, again for poorly understood reasons, include seizures, difficulties with sleep, and gastrointestinal (GI) disturbances. Although much remains to be learned, as we'll discuss later in this book, these medical conditions have recently provided new clues to causes of ASD. For example, epilepsy is diagnosed in a striking 20% of children with ASD—many times its incidence in the general population. This led to the interesting finding that many of the same genes implicated in ASD are implicated in epilepsy. For example, the gene *SCN2A* is the instruction manual for the production of a protein embedded in the walls of our brain cells that controls the passage of ions across the cell wall. That passage of ions across the cell wall is what dictates how a cell functions and communicates. Disruption of the gene *SCN2A* can either facilitate too much of the passage of ions or too little. It turns out that *too much* passage of the ions leads to epilepsy early in development, while *too little* leads to seizures later in development—and ASD.

Sleep problems are common in ASD. Over half of parents of children with ASD report their child has had some sort of sleep problem, and one-fourth of parents report their child does not get enough sleep. That sleep problems commonly occur in ASD is nothing new to parents, who have been talking to their doctors for years about these challenges. However, recent scientific advances have shown that behavioral interventions to improve sleep hygiene have significant effects on learning and reduction of problematic behaviors. We'll discuss those practical sleep improvement techniques in Chapter 6. And further, improvements in your child's sleep have a positive impact on your ability to sleep as well.

Silvia's school-age daughter struggled with sleep, and their family was receiving support from a sleep specialist. Silvia's daughter had autism and intellectual disability and had experienced significant sleep problems all of her life. She would sleep for only a couple of hours each night and would sometimes go for a day or two without any sleep, which interfered with the sleep of everyone else in the family as well. In the weeks following the sleep intervention, which included a combination of behavioral training and a prescription of melatonin, Silvia became less pale, the vibrancy of her hazel eyes emerged from under baggy eyelids, and even her posture was far straighter. She said that she had forgotten after 9 years what it was like to sleep a full night through. She felt revived and engaged in the world as she hadn't in nearly two decades. Sleep interventions that have been adapted for individuals with autism can be very effective, and the positive effects extend beyond simply a good night's sleep for your child.

Similar to sleep, gastrointestinal problems are common in ASD. It turns out this is not a coincidence but a powerful clue into the causes of autism. We talk about GI problems in depth in Chapter 7. Just to give a preview, we are now making rapid progress in understanding the relationship between GI problems and autism. This has led to a rapid change in clinical practice. Until recently, clinicians typically dismissed GI complaints as only of secondary or incidental concern. You may be among the parents who were told "We need to focus on the autism" or "I'm not sure what we can do about that." However, it has become clear that GI complaints significantly impact behavior—children with GI complaints have more problematic and challenging behavior than those who don't. And that makes sense. If you're uncomfortable or in pain, surmountable stresses or frustrations can quickly become insurmountable. Over time the medical community has taken parents' comments to heart, and now GI interventions for children with GI problems are incorporated into treatment plans.

In summary, intellectual and language impairments, ADHD, sleep, GI problems, and other associated conditions both complicate the planning for your child and provide usable scientific clues that we will turn into practical tips as we go through this book. The goal is enabling you to more readily create the "just right" individual plan for your child.

AUTISM CAN BE DIAGNOSED EARLIER THAN WE THOUGHT

One of the first questions you likely heard from your doctor was "When did you first become concerned?" The answer to this question will vary for different parents and children. As surprising as it may seem, as recently as the late 1980s, ASD wasn't diagnosed with confidence until late preschool age or even middle childhood. Clinicians simply did not know much about the early manifestations of autism. That changed with groundbreaking studies conducted in the 1990s, again emerging from parent–scientist collaborations, revealing that autism symptoms actually could be detected before the first birthday. However, it takes time to translate these scientific advances to the community, which is why there is a lag from scientific understanding to clinical practices that are available to families. As a result, it has only been in the past decade that we've seen clinicians apply this information to practice.

These first studies, conducted by one of us (Dawson) 25 years ago, broke new ground. The scientists obtained first-birthday videotapes from parents of school-age children definitively diagnosed with autism; they compared these to past videotapes of school-age children who developed in a typical manner without autism. The first birthday party just happened to provide something scientists prize greatly: a fairly standardized context in which to observe behavior. Most first birthday parties at some point have the child seated at a table, with friends and family gathered around. Typically, singing begins, a cake topped with flames or candles appears, and then there is lots of clapping. The tapes were coded by college students who had no idea which children had later developed autism. They were trained to simply rate the frequency of basic social behaviors, such as making eye contact or looking at faces. Although the first studies were very small, just a few key behaviors provided excellent (though not perfect) accuracy in separating which children would subsequently be diagnosed with ASD and which children would not: looking toward a person who said their name, the use of gestures, such as pointing and showing, and how much attention they paid to the people at the party (i.e., how much they looked at them). This study, and others like it, demonstrated that autism begins to emerge very early in life and pointed to behaviors clinicians might use for early screening and diagnosis. This opened the potential for imagining early intervention as an approach to prevent full development of ASD when the brain is most "plastic" (or responsive to input) in its formation. That, in turn, has provided new hope for the effectiveness of early intervention. More on this in Chapter 4.

But other recent discoveries complicate the picture. It's not just that social skills are absent in early development. In fact, quite the contrary. Most often, babies who will later develop autism usually start out by making normal eye contact, responding normally to having their name called, and paying typical attention to other people. Then, between about 6 and 8 months, they diverge: they begin to subtly and gradually pay less and less attention to people. For some infants, however, symptoms are not pronounced until 12 months or even older. These new findings indicate that development starts typically but changes in early infancy.

This early "regression" or departure from the expected social development route seems to be the norm in autism, rather than the exception.

Usually, it occurs during the first year. However, providing another important clue to our puzzle, in a minority of children who will develop autism, that regression happens around 18–24 months of age. This can occur either gradually or fairly rapidly. This pattern can include loss of previously acquired language and social skills or simply a failure to progress or a plateau in development.

By studying the very early development of infants later diagnosed with ASD, we have learned that the early course and pattern of symptom onset are quite variable across children. We have also discovered that infants later diagnosed with ASD show other early symptoms, such as difficulties with feeding, sleep, and motor development. And some children end up with only very mild ASD symptoms, while others require lifelong supports. By the time a child is 18–24 months old, however, the *diagnosis* of autism tends to be stable for the majority of children.

SOME CHILDREN LOSE THE DIAGNOSIS

Some features may emerge in the first year (although many diagnostic errors will still occur at that age), and the ASD diagnosis may be confidently made by about age 2, yet even then it's important to note that all children show at least some improvement once they begin to receive therapy. In addition, perhaps as many as 10% lose their autism symptoms altogether by school age—although those children typically show some other neurodevelopmental difficulty, such as ADHD, or emotional challenge, such as anxiety, that presumably led to the "false positive" in early life. When a child is very young—in the first 2 years of life—it is impossible to know whether the child's autism will end up being mild or severe. The important point is that you'll want to do what you can to help your individual child reach her full potential.

One driver for improving your child's outcome is early intervention—an exciting discovery. As we'll discuss later in this book, behaviorally based interventions for autism now bring great excitement because they really do work. However, they can be costly and difficult to obtain—in later chapters we'll explore some new ideas to build on this progress depending on your situation.

The Sex-Ratio Gap Is Narrower Than Once Believed

Autism is diagnosed in boys four times more often than it is diagnosed in girls. One speculation was that this was due to genetic mutations linked to sex chromosomes, but it's become increasingly clear that it's not this simple. Rather, on the genetic side recent discoveries indicate that females with ASD tend to have higher rates of rare genetic mutations, or variants (discussed more in Chapter 3), than males with autism, but these variants are scattered throughout the entire set of genes (the genome) and not linked to the sex chromosomes. In fact, when looking at children with ASD who have these rare mutations, the sex ratio drops from 4:1 to closer to 1:1. Moreover, some rare gene variants that mothers pass on to their sons and daughters seem to cause ASD only in the boys and not the girls. These findings are interesting for two reasons. One is that the findings are consistent with the theory of female protection (that it is harder for girls to get ASD); in other words, for a girl to develop autism she needs more genetic disruption than a boy does. This "female protective factor" related to ASD is also seen in some other brain development disorders and may be related to how sex hormones differentially influence brain development in boys and girls prenatally. The other reason is that it adds to the idea there are multiple routes to ASD—rare genetic mutations are one route, and boys seem more sensitive to a given number of these mutations. The other, possibly more common routes likely involve complex mixtures of genes and environments, as we'll discuss throughout the book.

New advances in our understanding also suggest that autism looks different in the brain of each sex and may also produce different behavior in girls. That is, given the same underlying cause of ASD, the behaviors may look different or be milder in girls than in boys.

New research also suggests that autism is more often missed or misdiagnosed in girls—perhaps because clinicians expect it more in boys or due to other differences in how girls and boys with ASD behave—and that this accounts, at least in part, for the 4:1 sex ratio in ASD. The specific symptoms that girls exhibit might differ in how they are expressed or their severity. Some studies suggest that girls are better at "camouflaging" their symptoms compared to boys. The implications here are that we need to pay closer attention to subtle behavioral challenges to make sure we're not missing diagnoses in girls with ASD.

WHAT KIND OF "SCIENCE" DO WE USE TO INCREASE OUR UNDERSTANDING OF ASD?

Throughout this book we'll be discussing findings from recent scientific advances in autism. We'll be extracting the key concepts and findings from different types of scientific studies. Each of these kinds of studies has strengths and weaknesses and offers pieces of the puzzle that we aim to integrate for you throughout this book. We highlight several of those study designs in the box on pages 24–25, so that as you review new findings that emerge in the scientific literature you have a little background as to the basis for our suggestions. We've pulled together the findings from all types of approaches, from meta-analyses to randomized controlled trials and prospective studies, to provide you with what the new science tells us about autism and, most important, what steps you can take toward making the changes that work best for your family.

WHERE DOES OUR NEW UNDERSTANDING OF ASD LEAVE CHILDREN—AND PARENTS?

Increased awareness and the new science of autism have raised questions about how to think about ASD. One question is philosophical—what is autism? Is it a disorder to be treated or a natural variation in development to be appreciated, or both? Many family members and the providers involved in care for individuals with ASD aim to intervene to reduce or minimize the core symptoms that define ASD to enhance the opportunity for that child to shape his own destiny and achieve his own potential. For example, if a child exhibits repetitive behaviors, such as making unusual motor movements, a goal of treatment might be to reduce the frequency of such movements and provide the child with greater flexibility in behavior choices.

However, as in all of psychiatry, it's crucial to distinguish "helping someone achieve her true potential" from "moving someone toward conformity to social norms." Sensitive to this risk, many advocate viewing ASD as representing differences that are part of the natural variation in ways of being human, a position that favors a focus on celebrating

Different Types of Scientific Research Studies

• *Meta-analysis.* A meta-analysis is an approach in which all studies that address a common question are combined into one analysis to draw strong conclusions about that question. This approach, when done well, overcomes the problem that single studies are prone to chance findings, particularly if they have small samples. The meta-analysis greatly increases confidence in the estimation of an effect because it can better adjust for chance findings in individual studies. One common use of meta-analyses is to determine the degree of effectiveness of a treatment. Now, just as individual study results are less reliable if they are small or used weak methods, the reliability of a meta-analysis also depends on the size, quality, and number of individual studies being reviewed. That said, generally the findings will provide more definitive understanding of a topic than the insights from a single study.

• *Systematic review.* Systematic reviews are similar to meta-analytic studies in that they pull together the entire literature on a question using rigorous rules, but they provide less insight into the quantitative effect of a given intervention or variable under study. However, like meta-analyses, they pull together key findings from across studies, illuminating patterns that any single study cannot.

• *Randomized controlled trials.* Randomized controlled trials are a powerful way to isolate and examine the effect of a treatment. Their power comes from randomly assigning people to either a treatment group or a placebo group. When done well, the placebo is disguised so expectations from the participants or the experimenters cannot bias the results. The power of randomization is statistical—it means that when the study succeeds, we know for sure that the treatment caused the improvement and that the improvement is not due to some unmeasured factor in the situation. The treatment being studied can be anything from a 2-year behavioral intervention to a 6-week dietary approach to a single dose of medication. In this type of "double-blind" study (meaning neither the scientist nor the study subjects know which group each person is in) any conscious or unconscious biases that anyone involved in the study may have can be ruled out. The randomization also allows for ruling out any other systematic differences that could influence the results. The key strength of this type of experimental design is that it can show that one thing caused another, not merely that the two just happened to appear together, which is what correlational studies demonstrate.

• *Prospective studies.* To improve our understanding of what autism looked like during early development scientists relied on retrospective studies, reviews of events and information that happened in the past. More recently, prospective studies have been used to shed light on autism. In prospective studies individuals with autism are followed over a period of time. These studies are important because an earlier event or "risk factor" is a clue to a cause and because they help us predict what might happen for different children even when we aren't sure of the cause. For example, in a prospective study younger siblings of a child with autism (who we know are more likely to develop autism than the population at large) may be followed from birth and their patterns of behavior or exposure to experiences measured. Then some years later they can be assessed for ASD, and those earlier measurements can perhaps inform or predict diagnostic outcomes. While this type of study design would not prove causation, it is still more powerful than simply looking at the presence of behaviors and ASD symptoms at a single point in time. In that case we wouldn't be able to determine which came first.

• *Whole-population studies.* Large population-based studies have proven invaluable in examining links between exposures and autism or the presence of genetic factors and autism because they can detect subtle effects that a smaller study would miss. In most studies of autism, participants are recruited from the local community or a clinic. This local approach has the advantage that kids can be evaluated in depth. But it has the disadvantage that results may not generalize to the whole population of children with ASD. Computing power and large databases have allowed scientists to examine data from much larger groups of individuals with autism, thereby increasing the likelihood that findings could be generalized to all individuals with autism. Their disadvantage is that the individuals cannot be assessed in depth, so there may be diagnostic errors and other limitations.

neurodiversity. Thus, they encourage efforts to focus on acceptance of ASD and reduce any disability associated with ASD by adapting the environment. People with this perspective might ask, "What is wrong with making unusual motor movements, especially if such movements help the child or adult feel less stressed? We should help other people accept these differences unless they are causing harm."

The idea that autism is a difference that should be accepted has been championed by many, including adults with autism, or autistic people, which is the term that some self-advocates would prefer to use. This perspective is particularly important when individuals are already functioning quite well—for example, many of these adults are able to engage with the community and succeed in a variety of settings as part of everyday life, although not without challenges associated with ASD, such as sensory sensitivities or difficulty understanding social cues. These individuals don't want their challenges to be misunderstood by others, and thus they advocate for increased acceptance of the differences that are part of ASD, as well as whatever supports are needed to succeed. What we call ASD is experienced as part of their personality and identity—not something they want "healed."

At the same time, many people with ASD are suffering considerably. They are not able to engage in the broader community without significant treatment and support, such as having a constant caregiver and augmentative communication devices, which makes them vulnerable to serious suffering should those supports not be obtainable. Increasing their capacity to care for themselves and make their own informed decisions by increasing their skills is thus seen as a vital goal by many individuals, families, and caregivers as well as the mental health treatment community.

How you end up thinking about your child's autism (and how your child will ultimately think about it) will be a personal decision, which will likely be influenced by the nature of your child's autism, as well as personal and cultural perspectives. Science cannot provide a definitive answer to the value questions here. There is no "right" or "wrong" answer. Your view of autism will be shaped by your and your child's individual experience. Regardless, your caring, accepting, and encouraging attitude toward your child will help your child and others feel valued and more confident.

So, as a parent, what can you do with this new understanding of autism? The first thing you can do is recognize that because autism falls on a spectrum, each child has unique challenges and strengths and thus interventions and supports will be individualized. Autism is not a "one-intervention-fits-all" type of diagnosis. One child may benefit from an intensive one-on-one treatment plan, whereas another may be better served in a group setting. One child may benefit from speech therapy, whereas another child may want to speak incessantly. The notion of a unique treatment and intervention plan can seem overwhelming at first, but recent scientific advances have provided a road map for developing a unique plan for moving forward with your child. That road map will include components from the latest scientific evidence outlining what is helpful, will include supports that build on your child's strengths while addressing your child's challenges, and will incorporate measures to manage co-occurring medical concerns. The second step you can take, given our new understanding of autism, is to educate yourself on what the science tells us about what autism is, how children develop, and what we can do to help each child with autism live the life that he or she wants to live. That step will provide you with the knowledge you need to sift through all the information and misinformation that is out there. It will also help you understand how your child thinks. By understanding how your child learns and thrives you will be in the best position to support him. Your third step will be to put together your own road map based on this information that you've pulled together about what autism is and what kinds of help can be included in a treatment package. This is a time to be hopeful. So let's get started.

2

WHAT ARE THE ESSENTIAL FEATURES THAT DEFINE THE AUTISM SPECTRUM?

We focused on the significant differences among individuals with autism in Chapter 1 because understanding that autism falls along a spectrum is essential to getting the best outcome for any individual child. But it's also important to know what all individuals with autism have in common. What do we consider the "essence" of autism? What are the features that are shared by individuals, accounting for the fact that these children are all viewed as part of one spectrum? DSM-5 lists the basic characteristics that define autism as falling into two categories: (1) impairments in social communication and interaction and (2) the presence of restricted and repetitive interests and behaviors. If your child is on the spectrum, you are undoubtedly familiar with the outward signs of these characteristics. But unpacking them to gain an understanding of what is going on in the mind and brain of your child that produces these characteristics can shed a lot more light on how to help the child.

IMPAIRMENTS IN SOCIAL DEVELOPMENT

There are two key elements that help explain why children with autism have difficulties relating socially to others. One has to do with how interested your child is in the social world, referred to as "social motivation."

In general, those with autism tend to be less interested in and pay less attention to social information. Social information has lower value for them. The second element is the ability to process or make sense of social information, such as the ability to accurately read social cues like facial expressions. A combination of clever observational and brain imaging studies from the past 10 years has built a clearer picture of how the mind works differently in autism with regard to these two critical components of social engagement. And while in theory each could drive the other, for a couple of reasons we favor the belief that social motivation is key and can contribute to difficulties in social information processing. One reason is that working from that perspective has led to effective ways to help children with ASD. Another is information we've obtained from studies of brain activity.

Differences in Social Motivation

Let's start with the classic picture. When Leo Kanner first described ASD, he presented 11 case studies of children he had seen in his clinic. He described one child as having "a disinclination to play with children and do things children his age usually take an interest in doing." He described a second child by referring to his mother's statements, for example, "he mostly ignored other people. When we had guests, he just wouldn't pay any attention." Similarly, for a third child, Kanner reported, "he showed no interest in the examiner or any other person." For all the children in his pioneering case reports he mentioned the reduced attention to the social world.

Here's a fairly simple way that scientists initially nailed down this element of autism: Picture an empty room with a simple table in the center. Seated at the table is a toddler with ASD, and sitting opposite is a graduate student. Together they are quietly playing with Play-Doh. Periodically, from four precisely designated locations, two diagonally behind the child and two diagonally behind the graduate student, a second graduate student presents different types of sounds all at the same volume. These include common sounds such as a kitchen timer, an alarm clock, and a car horn, representing nonsocial sounds, and also hands clapping, a voice calling the child's name, and thigh slapping, representing social sounds. A third experimenter, watching from behind a one-way mirror, is counting the number of times the child pays attention to the various sounds. This basic experiment was repeated with placement of the sounds around the room and the order of the presentation alternated and balanced to control for the influence of location or order for dozens of children with ASD, children with developmental delay, and children with typical development. When the number of turns toward the sounds was added up across all the children, the toddlers with ASD had paid attention to the social stimuli far less than their toddler peers—and this seems to be true for everyone with autism, cutting across all the many differences discussed in Chapter 1.

But isn't that approach error prone? After all, it relies on human actors and coders. To confirm this observation, new technologies have gone further. By hijacking the same eye-tracking technology that air force pilots use to identify and track targets when rocketing across the sky, scientists now can use specially calibrated cameras and complicated mathematical algorithms to track where children with ASD look at all times when presented with static and dynamic images on video screens. A striking finding here emerges when individuals with autism view pictures and movies involving human faces. Those with ASD attend to the face—but not the same part of the face as other children. Most typically developing children in this situation focus mainly on the eyes. We think this is because the eyes convey the most information about what the other person is noticing and feeling. Children with ASD tend to look at the eyes no more often than any other part of the face. They may look at the chin or the mouth just as often. Although not literally true, it is almost as if the face appears to them as a complex geometric shape, rather than a face. In a room containing a variety of objects as well as people, typically developing children will focus most of their attention on the people, but children with ASD may spend just as much time looking at the objects in the room. Why might this be? Both low social motivation and impairments in social information processing likely are at play. Which came first may be a chicken-and-egg situation.

What Is Going On in the Brain?

One reason we suspect low social motivation is primary, however, is that brain imaging studies with individuals with autism tend to find reduced activity in parts of the brain that support motivation—especially when the motivation is social in nature.

Scientists have used structural magnetic resonance imaging (MRI) to examine the size and shape of the structures in the brain and functional magnetic resonance imaging (fMRI) to examine what parts of the brain are active when a person is engaged in a task. Greater brain activity is inferred based on how much blood is flowing to a particular part of the brain during an activity. Based on measures of both structural and functional MRI, we have learned that the brain of a person with ASD is different. This difference involves the complex interplay between different structures and regions including the amygdala, an almond-shaped structure nestled deep within our brains; the ventral striatum, located above the amygdala but still below the cortical layer of our brain; and regions of the most evolutionarily advanced part of our brains, the prefrontal cortex. The amygdala tags information as salient and biologically relevant to us, alerting us to attend to those things critical to our survival.

For example, when you're wandering through the woods in your local park and you stumble across a snake sunning itself along the trail, your startle response is the result, in part, of your amygdala telling you to attend to this object in your path. The amygdala is tightly connected to the ventral striatum, which is a part of the brain that is active during rewarding activities—everything ranging from falling in love to inhaling cocaine, as well as relatively commonplace activities like receiving social praise for a job well done. The orbitofrontal cortex, which has dense connections to the amygdala and ventral striatum, is largely involved in integrating the inputs from the amygdala and ventral striatum to guide goal-directed action and respond to changing feedback from the environment.

In ASD, on average, the amygdala differs in size (is larger in some studies and smaller in others), has atypical connections with other brain structures, and shows reduced activity when responding to pictures of social stimuli, such as faces and eyes. (These brain changes are small and too subtle to see in an individual child, at least with today's technology, so no, there is not a brain scan test for ASD at this point.) In the same vein, when performing tasks where the reward is either social in nature, such as receiving praise from a charismatic undergraduate student, or nonsocial in nature, such as receiving a monetary prize, individuals with ASD on average show decreased activity in the ventral striatum during social rewards but normal levels of activity of these reward circuits when the reward is an object of interest to the person. Thus, the motivational element altered here seems to be specific to social information, not motivation in general, based on the brain scan studies. What appears to be happening in the ASD brain is that social stimuli are not tagged as salient, and thus the neural circuits that assign reward to faces, voices, gestures, and other social stimuli are not activated.

> The brains of children with autism seem to be wired to make them less motivated by the social aspects of their world than typical children.

It is not hard to imagine then, if a child's brain does not tag social information as noteworthy or motivating from very early on in life, that the child won't attend to those stimuli during development. If the child is not attending to social stimuli, like faces or eyes or interactions between two people, that child will miss out on the rich tapestry of information specific to our social world, like how to interpret emotional expressions, how to respond to questions, how to greet someone, and how to have a conversation. Gradually, the child will fail to gain or will lose the ability even to accurately read social information like facial expressions. This is why some infants and toddlers may appear to be developing typically at first: It's only after the lost opportunities to learn socially begin to add up to produce observable symptoms that they are diagnosed.

Here's an analogy that may be helpful. Imagine one of us (Bernier), as a clinical researcher, doesn't find football motivating. I naturally ignore sports news and tend to "tune out" when conversations turn to football. As a result, now I miss out on all the cues and information that football conversations reveal, including the basics like the rules of the game and who is playing—and even when I do see that information, I have nowhere in my mind to store it, so I fail to appreciate its importance. However, encouragement from a friend to memorize the rules of the game and see some games creates a different dynamic. Now, knowing something about the game and attending games with a friend who makes it fun, I find it is interesting—and as a result, I learn more by attending to it. Finally, through the association of the good experiences with the friend, my motivation to learn about football increases even more. This silly "friend" intervention example results in improved football knowledge in the same way that behaviorally based interventions can improve social motivation and social processing in a "virtuous cycle" for kids with ASD. That is, the reverse pattern can work as well. Imagine a child who doesn't engage in social interactions but loves football. We can use that child's love of football to promote social opportunities and provide social experiences where social skills can be practiced and developed, and over time the associations with the reward of football can be linked to social interactions.

Integrating a child's special interest into social interactions can provide opportunities to improve social motivation and social processing.

Despite the fact that most children with autism showed reduced interest in social information, many are nevertheless affectionate and enjoy being with people. Many children enjoy sharing their special interests with others, as well as activities such as rough-and-tumble play and musical games. Spending time with your child performing the child's preferred activities is a good way to increase your child's motivation and interest in others.

Differences in Social Information Processing

By increasing a child's motivation to attend to social information, we can improve social information processing, the brain's ability to interpret cues from the social world and make sense of that information. One simple example highlighting how behavioral interventions can lead to increased attention to social information concerns efforts to increase eye contact. Making eye contact is critical for learning about the social world. One way to teach eye contact is to encourage it by rewarding it. Let's say a child loves bubbles but doesn't make good eye contact. An interventionist working on eye contact could hold the bubble container next to her own face. When the child (accidentally or intentionally) makes eye contact, the interventionist immediately rewards the eye contact by blowing some bubbles. That pairing of the bubbles with the eye contact is repeated over and over. And, over time, the interventionist can increase the distance between the bubble container and her face but still reward the eye contact with bubble blowing. Again, over hundreds of such pairings the child learns to pair that social interaction, eye contact, with rewards and can then begin to use it to facilitate communication (e.g., "I'd like some bubbles, please").

However, paying attention to the social world is not enough. Even children who start to pay attention to the social world may find social information difficult to process at times. Social information, such as talking and expressing emotions, is inherently complex, ever changing and unpredictable, and multisensory. Science has shown that the parts of the brain used to process social information, conveniently termed the "social brain," are different in ASD, and this helps explain how children with ASD process (or fail to process) important social cues.

> By making the social world more rewarding so that your child is more likely to attend to social information, you can provide more opportunities to learn about the social world, but it may not be enough, since the social world is so complex.

The social world is dynamic, challenging, and fast paced. Consider the complexities in a simple greeting from a bus driver to a child going to school for the day. The bus pulls up to the bus stop, and there are a dozen faces, all with different expressions, peering out from the windows and a dozen more faces partly obscured by looking every which way inside the bus. There are no fewer than a score of differing vocalizations ranging in tone, pitch, frequency, and pace emanating from the yellow bus. These sounds have to be disentangled from the rumbling of the engine and the hiss of the brakes while the additional inputs to the sensory experience, like the smell of the diesel fuel and the wafting of the warm air from the radiator, have to be tuned out as well. The door opens, and from the driver's seat atop the stairs the driver calls, "C'mon in, Raphe; I haven't got all day" as she points to the back of the bus with her hooked thumb. At the same time her eyebrows are creased, her nose is scrunched, her lips are tight and thin. The actual words she says need to be heard and interpreted and mapped against both her facial expressions and her body language. This short message needs to be siphoned from the rest of the sounds and sights in the bus and considered in the context of the activity, in this case heading off to school for the day. All of this complex processing and interpretation has to happen quickly and in a rapidly shifting, dynamic interaction. For most individuals, learning to do this is "automatic"—kids just kind of pick it up by osmosis, the same way they learn a language by being around it. But in ASD, that doesn't happen.

You can imagine that if it's not automatic the welter of such social information quickly becomes overwhelming to try to process.

Face Recognition

Recent research suggests that, similar to challenges with social motivation, difficulties with processing social information are central to ASD. One striking piece of evidence that has emerged in the past 10 years comes from recording electrical signals from the brain using harmless electrodes (detectors) on the scalp. In typically developing individuals, this method reveals that people recognize a face as being, in fact, a face and not something else, within less than 200 milliseconds—just a fraction of a second! This is almost as fast as conscious awareness itself. The brain has developed a specialized pattern-recognition ability to recognize human faces as being human faces. In individuals with autism, this recognition takes longer, suggesting a subtle but important weakness in the brain's face recognition system.

However, there's a wrinkle: if an individual with ASD is instructed to pay attention to the faces (and aided with a visual cue as to where the face will appear), that delay is mostly eliminated. This highlights that some combination of motivation (attending to faces as relevant) and processing (recognizing faces as faces quickly enough) is involved in autism. The good news is that heartening findings like this point the way to behavioral training that can help children with ASD "grow" their face-processing ability. And they indicate that directing a child's attention to faces improves his ability to process that face. So, by reinforcing attention to faces, as in our bubble-blowing example above, we can increase attention to faces. This should, in theory, create a "virtuous cycle" as the child attends to a face more often and then reaps the positive benefits of doing so.

Biological Motion

Faces are obviously pivotal to our social life. But they are just as clearly not the whole story. Other kinds of information processing are also crucial to the brain's social-information-processing abilities. Another part of the story is what scientists call "biological motion." Biological motion means movements that are characteristic of living animals and, more particularly, human and socially meaningful—walking, dancing, reaching out a hand to shake it, or performing impressive kung fu moves (this last one, however, is not in our repertoire). Just as the brain has dedicated modules for processing faces, scientists have recently discovered that it also has a distinct module (a part of the temporal lobe) specialized for processing biological motion.

This discovery was made using what are called point-light displays. These are like cartoons: they are essentially movies in which points of light are shown against a black background, either depicting everyday movements like riding a bicycle or randomly careening across the screen, but there are no actual people (or animals) depicted—just patterns of moving dots. Remarkably, most people quickly recognize human-like patterns of movement versus other patterns. When this experiment is done using MRI, scientists can identify specific activity in a brain circuit anchored in an area called the brain's superior temporal sulcus (STS). Brain activity in this area is reduced in individuals with ASD. But similar to the findings in face processing, there is good news here. As we'll discuss in Chapter 3, brain activity in this region apparently can be normalized through practice, once again indicating promise for treatment approaches targeting social difficulties in individuals with ASD.

> When we know where activity in the brain is different in those with ASD, we can design interventions that shift that activity toward normal through behavioral practice—like paying attention to and recognizing human faces.

Theory of Mind

A third key part of the brain's ability to process social information is referred to as "theory of mind"—the capacity to understand that other people have thoughts and feelings that are distinct from one's own. A story used for now-classic studies with children involves three children; we'll call them Josh, Anne, and Olivia. Josh has placed a marble in one of two baskets. His friend Anne watched Josh put that marble in the basket on the left. Anne then leaves, and unbeknown to Anne (and for reasons that will remain mysterious), Josh moves the marble to the basket on the right. Olivia has been watching this activity and sees him do this. Now Anne returns to retrieve her marble. Olivia is asked, "Where do you think she'll look?" Of course, you, the reader, know that Anne will look for the marble in the basket on the left, where she saw Josh place it. Typically developing children also know this by a young age. The reason you (and most children) can know this is that you have developed a *theory of mind*. That's a fancy way of saying that you recognize implicitly that Anne has her own perceptions distinct from your own; therefore, Anne will act on the basis of her own beliefs and knowledge, not yours. This ability comes online in typically developing children around 4½ years of age. Younger preschoolers and toddlers will respond that Anne will look for the marble in the basket to the right because that's where the marble is, and they know that's where it is, and so therefore they believe Anne will, too—they don't yet understand that others have different perspectives from their own. The same is true of many children over age 5 on the autism spectrum. If Olivia has ASD, she may say that Anne will look in the basket on the right even if Olivia is 8. Very young children and kids on the spectrum will also have difficulty understanding games such as hide-and-seek, which require an understanding of theory of mind. Even lying requires a theory of mind and, not surprisingly, many people with autism don't engage in lying. This is a wonderful characteristic in most situations. However, the ability to tell "white lies" helps us navigate many social situations, such as when Aunt Mary asks whether you like her funny-looking hat.

Even though individuals with ASD struggle with tasks like this long after the age of 5, many of them can learn to complete this task accurately over the course of their development. Many children with ASD are able to reason out the appropriate answer using concrete logic without relying on a theory of mind, but for other children with ASD, social experience might drive the development of the ability to correctly complete these types of tasks.

While the Josh–Anne–Olivia task is easy for teens and adults with ASD, theory of mind is still not typical even in adults with ASD. This difficulty is identified using age-appropriate tests for adults. One task is called "Reading the Mind in the Eyes." In this test, you see a series of pictures of faces with only a sliver of the face—the eyes—visible. Surrounding each pair of eyes are four emotion words like "distrustful," "jealous," "panicked," and "angry." You have to select the word that best characterizes the emotion in the eyes. It sounds hard, but in fact, most adults can easily do this. In contrast, adults with ASD tend to have difficulty on this task and be less accurate than most other people.

Brain imaging using MRI suggests that our "social brain" uses a brain area called the temporo-parietal junction (for neuroscientists, this is such a famous and important area for social function, for attention, and other abilities that it is just referred to in affectionate shorthand as the TPJ). The TPJ is close to the STS, which as we explained earlier is involved in processing biological motion. As one lighthearted study revealed, when British adults with ASD were asked to estimate how likely it was for the British queen to think that keeping a diary is important, they showed reduced activation in this region. Typical adults showed activation of the TPJ in response to this question because of the requirement that a reader not only consider another person's perspective but also

---

How DSM-5 Lowers the Risk of Overdiagnosing Autism

Social communication and interaction deficits are central to the diagnosis of ASD as provided in DSM-5. That's why DSM-5 requires children to demonstrate deficits in all of the listed domains of social challenges (social reciprocity, nonverbal communication, and relationships) to be diagnosed with ASD. The fourth edition of the DSM inadvertently created opportunities for overdiagnosis by including these challenges but spreading them across social impairments and language deficits. This fifth edition makes the criteria more reflective of current thinking about autism and more accurate because the criteria restrict the ability to "count" a deficit more than once, which could result in overdiagnosis. In DSM-IV, a clinician could, for example, cite challenges with conversation in the language domain (deficits in conversations) and the social domain (deficits in social reciprocity) and end up concluding that the child was at a more severe point on the spectrum than was actually the case and therefore should be diagnosed.

consider the perspective of a person who was not very relatable to the average British citizen.

What do the marble test, the mysterious eyes test, and related studies like this tell us about ASD? As you probably have guessed, they reveal that people with autism often find it challenging to understand what another person is thinking, feeling, and intending. This is clearly going to affect their social responses and sometimes make them seem "off." Thus, if your son with ASD fails to offer you a Kleenex or give you a hug when you are sad, it's not due to malice, coldness, or indifference, but rather a simple lack of processing or understanding. If your daughter fails to appropriately respond to small talk from the cashier at the grocery, it's probably because she doesn't understand why that cashier is talking to her or what the implicit intention of the cashier (to be friendly) really is. Fortunately, many individuals with autism do learn how to pay attention and understand the social world. Many well-studied behavioral therapies can help teach concepts such as emotions and perspective taking.

> *Social responses that may seem "off" can often be traced to the fact that those with ASD don't fully understand what others are thinking or feeling—they lack what we call a "theory of mind."*

RESTRICTED AND REPETITIVE INTERESTS AND BEHAVIORS

The social brain is obviously a major part of the story of autism today, and we now have a fairly deep understanding of the social brain that we did not have just 10 years ago. This has opened up exciting possibilities for helping children with ASD achieve their goals and potential. Information-processing styles in ASD also extend beyond social information, however, as you are no doubt aware. The second domain that is at the core of diagnosing of ASD concerns restricted and repetitive interests and behaviors. It's important to understand that a range of behaviors and differences related to overfocused interests (or inflexible thinking) fall under this domain, and not all children with ASD manifest all of them. This is why DSM-5 requires the presence of only two out of four of the domains of restricted or repetitive behaviors discussed below for an autism diagnosis.

In his classic descriptive study, Kanner described Case 10 like this: "Daily routine must be adhered to rigidly; any slightest change of the pattern called forth outbursts of panic. . . . He was extremely upset upon seeing anything broken or incomplete. He noticed two dolls to which he had paid no attention before. He saw that one of them had no hat and became very much agitated, wandering about the room to look for the hat. When the hat was retrieved from another room, he instantly lost all interest in the dolls." The way we view it today, this tendency to overfocus creates differences in four domains: the need for routine, stereotypic behaviors, narrow interests, and sensory sensitivities.

Inflexible Thinking and the Need for Sameness

Many of you will recognize this pattern in your own loved one with ASD. Kanner's young patient, "John," had tremendous difficulties with flexible thinking. The result was strict adherence to schedules, difficulty with transitions, and rigidity about how things were arranged. Subsequent to Kanner, scientists have noticed that beyond difficulties with transitions, inflexible thinking extends to difficulties in thinking abstractly. One parent told us, "Joey is just very concrete. If it's time to leave and I say, 'Let's hit the road,' he says, 'But that will hurt'—and he doesn't mean it as a joke!" The same difficulty is reflected in trouble imagining future plans or, more relevantly, adjusting when those plans are disrupted. This is why, even though it may seem trivial to us to one day detour for an errand on the way to the daily school drop-off, it is a really big deal for many kids with ASD. A total meltdown may follow. This is not necessarily your child being manipulative—it is that the child cannot process and make sense of what is happening, and so the situation quickly becomes overwhelming. His brain does not allow him to think flexibly, disengage from the current plans, and imagine a new plan for achieving the goal of going to school.

There is hope, however, in that recent discoveries are helping us understand this inflexibility of thinking or insistence on sameness. Several brain imaging studies in ASD have shown that the volume and density of neurons in parts of the brain that we've already mentioned, the striatum and the circuits of the brain that are closely linked to this region, including the prefrontal cortex, are different in individuals with

ASD. Similarly, functional imaging studies of the brain suggest reduced activity in these regions when individuals with ASD are performing tasks that require flexible thinking and inhibition of previously learned behaviors. This insight can point the way toward the development of new treatments that target those underlying brain circuits. We're not there yet, but understanding the neurobiology of complex behaviors like inflexible thinking is the first step.

Stereotypic Behaviors

"Stereotypic" essentially means repetitive, and stereotypic behaviors have been noted as part of ASD since Kanner's first description. These stereotypic behaviors include repetitive motor mannerisms, such as hand flapping or body posturing, and repetitive use of objects, such as lining up toys and picking up objects and repeatedly dropping them. Stereotyped behaviors also include repetitive speech patterns, such as scripted language. The scripted language can serve no obvious purpose, such as repeating back movie lines wherever and whenever, or it can be used functionally. For example, one child used the scripted phrase "time to get on the bus" any time he was ready to leave the room. That was his way of communicating his wishes. Unfortunately for one of us (Bernier), the child consistently said that every time we were in the room together. (I tried not to take it too personally.) Another example of stereotypic speech patterns is captured in the young man who had a range of interests, including Harry Potter. He was happy to share all sorts of facts about Legos, dinosaurs, and Pokemon as well. As he described these interests he used appropriate inflection, tone, and grammar, but the moment he switched topics to Harry Potter, he spoke with a British accent. However, he would seamlessly transition back to typical American inflections and intonation as he switched topics.

Interestingly, the same circuitry is disrupted in those with other disorders marked by repetitive behaviors, such as Tourette syndrome (a tic disorder in which the individual has an irresistible urge to repeat a movement or sound) and obsessive–compulsive disorder (characterized by irresistible urges to clean or double-check or count things). While the experiences of children with ASD are not the same as those of children with these disorders, they appear to be biologically related. As we learn more about the brain systems that suppress these urges or enable more flexibility, we gain an understanding that may yield new treatment ideas. We don't have any currently, but insight into the neurobiology provides new avenues for treatment exploration.

Narrow Interests

Narrow interests are also commonly observed in autism, although not all children with ASD have narrow interests. They can take two forms: interests that are unusual in their intensity and interests that are unusual in their focus. Interests that are unusual in their intensity, called circumscribed interests, are those interests that are like typical hobbies but become all-consuming for the child. That is, they might be all the child wants to talk about or play with to the detriment of social interactions or exposure to other experiences. One example would be the 13-year-old whose circumscribed interest was photography. Photography is a hobby that many individuals enjoy. For this young man, though, his interest got in the way of social interactions. He enjoyed sharing every fact about every camera that he knew, which was essentially the model number and year of production for every camera made. Another child I (Bernier) worked with had an intense interest in toilets. Upon entering a new building he would find all the toilets, examine them, note the brand, note the model, and share his findings with his parents. This is an example of what are termed unusual preoccupations—an interest in something that many would find unusual. Toilets, traffic lights, empty laundry detergent containers, and fire alarms are just a few of the examples that we've encountered in our clinical experiences.

Narrow interests can be difficult to negotiate in daily life, but they can also be channeled to serve vocational or academic interests.

Circumscribed interests and unusual preoccupations can have a significant impact on family life. Depending on the intensity of the interest, families may have to rearrange their daily lives to accommodate these interests or may have to manage meltdowns and tantrums if the interest cannot be pursued easily. These interests can also impede a child's ability to engage with others (who may tire of hearing facts about Pokemon characters) and engage in other activities outside that particular interest. On the other hand, special interests can be powerfully beneficial for the individual with ASD. If appropriately harnessed, special interests can serve vocational purposes. One might say that we, as academics, have narrow interests in the neurobiology of autism. We have been able to harness our intense interests in the service of advancing the field. But this isn't only true of academics. Microsoft has a program to hire and support individuals with ASD. One young man employed by Microsoft had an interest in computer coding and was able to use that interest to support his employment at Microsoft.

Additionally, narrow interests can be powerful reinforcers for helping us complete onerous tasks. I (Bernier) recall having an intense interest in mythical beasts as a school-age child. I loved to read about them, watch movies that featured them, draw pictures of them, and talk to my parents all about them. My parents used that interest to reward me for tackling my math homework (which in sixth grade I considered the most onerous task imaginable). The opportunity to watch a movie with my dad that involved the minotaur was something that kept me going throughout lengthy homework assignments. Knowledge of the reinforcing power of special interests has aided me in helping kids with ASD in school or in the clinic complete onerous tasks innumerable times. Recently, I used a child's interest in Lego Ninjago as a reinforcement to help him complete neuropsychological testing he needed to help guide his individualized education program (IEP) at his elementary school.

Sensory Processing

The boy who covers his ears with his hands when an ambulance races by, the girl who can't wear pants with a tag in the back, the child who will eat only white foods, and the young man who is distracted by the hum of the air conditioner that is imperceptible to the rest of us are all experiencing what clinical scientists call "sensory sensitivities." These examples capture what could be a hyperreactivity to the social world. That is, the child is hyperreactive to the sensory stimuli. Alternatively, the boy who runs his hands through the hair of everyone around him, including those on the subway seat next to him, the girl who puts everything she holds to her lips for a moment when she first grabs it, the young man who stares at all fans from the corner of his eye, and the child who regularly licks his neighbor's doorstep all have a related experience called "sensory interests." These are examples of hyporeactivity—the child underreacts to social stimuli and seeks out additional, and sometimes specific, experiences to stimulate the sensory experience. These features have long been controversial in autism research, with scientists debating their centrality. However, by 2013 the picture had become clear, and the presence of sensory sensitivities and/or interests was added to the official diagnostic criteria for autism in DSM-5. Indeed, it is striking that 95% of parents with a child on the spectrum will note some sort of hyporeactivity or hyperreactivity to sensory stimuli in that child.

Though DSM-5 lists sensory sensitivities under the core feature involving inflexible thinking (restricted, repetitive patterns of behavior, interests, or activities), we now know that sensory sensitivities and social processing difficulties are connected, a discovery supported by studies on mice. While it may sound strange to use a mouse to study autism, under certain conditions mice demonstrate behaviors that scientists think are similar enough to autistic behaviors in humans to teach us something useful. For example, when a certain gene called *MeCP2* is deactivated, mice engage in repetitive movements and demonstrate social problems (they spend less time with unfamiliar mice and do less sniffing, crawling over, or grooming with unfamiliar mice). Scientists think these behaviors are possibly related to what happens in people with autism. Researchers also conducted experiments in which some mice had a disruption to *MeCP2* only in brain cells, others only in the cells of their peripheral nervous system—the cells involved, say, in sensation on the skin or muscles in the leg. The mice with *MeCP2* disrupted ("knocked out") in brain cells showed behaviors like repetitive hind-limb clasping and motor challenges, but no sensitivities to touch. They also built nests for offspring, seemed to interact normally with other mice, and were the same as the other mice in their willingness to explore a maze or shake off the startle of a loud noise. In contrast, those mice with *MeCP2* knocked out peripherally were hypersensitive to touch, didn't adapt to loud noises, didn't interact with other mice or make nests for offspring, and didn't explore mazes. Yet they also had normal motor movement without any obvious repetitive movements. This study suggests that the same genetic differences can explain both sensory sensitivities and social development.

Scientists have conducted the same type of experiment on mice with disruptions to the gene *GABRB3,* with similar results. When the mice were hypersensitive to touch, social deficits followed. (However, the picture held only in developing mice; it was different for adult mice. We'll talk more about how ASD may change in development in Chapter 4.)

Other studies in people and in animals seem to converge in the following picture: While the need for sameness (repetition, routine) and difficulties with social processing seem to be distinct features of ASD, the sensory sensitivities in ASD seem to be somehow related to the social challenges. For example, studies show that sensory sensitivities in very early life are associated with later difficulties with language and social development. This could be partly due to interference with learning. A child who is sensitive to loud noises might retreat from situations with loud noises, like group activities or play, and without that experience and interaction she will miss out on the chance to practice and develop the social skills inherent in those scenarios— creating a kind of "vicious cycle."

> *Studies of mice have shown that both sensory sensitivities and problems in social development can be caused by the same genetic difference in ASD.*

Studies like these have identified a connection at both the molecular and behavioral levels between alterations in sensory and social information processing in ASD, as well as a developmental progression to this relationship, in which sensory sensitivities may interfere with social learning but might not do so when those sensitivities emerge later in life. This suggests that helping your child cope with sensory sensitivities may enhance treatment focusing on improving social skills. The key point for parents is that if you bring sensory sensitivities to the attention of your clinician as soon as they appear, they are likely to be addressed early, reducing the negative impact they may have on the development of your child's social skills.

Multisensory Processing

The connection between sensory problems and social deficits becomes even clearer when we consider the fact that children with ASD are not only vulnerable to sensory sensitivities but also have trouble connecting input from different senses and using that combined information to make decisions or draw conclusions. For example, some speech sounds that a person hears are impacted by what the listener is watching. This is called the McGurk illusion, in which a listener's experience of spoken words is unconsciously modified by what the listener sees the speaker articulating. Depending on how a speaker's mouth moves to articulate certain sounds, the listener will experience different sounds even when the same sound is heard. Interestingly, studies have shown that effects like the McGurk illusion are diminished in people with autism. That is, the listener with ASD is less impacted than others by the visual information in the experience of the speech sound. Similarly, for decades it has been noted that children and adults with ASD struggle with imitating actions such as facial expressions or hand gestures or personal mannerisms. The ability to imitate requires integration of visual stimuli and one's own body movements. If you have difficulty integrating what you see someone doing with how your body should move to re-create that action, you will struggle to accurately imitate it.

In our example from earlier in the chapter of the young man getting on the bus, it is clear that all the different stimuli need to be processed and integrated. If components of that processing are delayed or attended to more or less relative to other stimuli, then the seamless and easy multimodal integration is neither seamless nor easy. In fact it can feel quite overwhelming, like the way a tired adult feels in a crowded airport hearing an announcement that the gate has changed and boarding is now beginning—and the new gate is a half-hour walk away. The result is that he feels confused and overwhelmed (which in children translates to "meltdown" and in children with ASD to "getting stuck").

From that example you can infer that if sensory experiences aren't integrating well, then the social world gets particularly overwhelming and hard to handle. It's not hard to imagine that children with ASD might avoid social situations, leading to delays in the development of social skills. Again, this points to the importance of addressing those sensory challenges to improve social deficits and ultimately the quality of life for your child. Fortunately, we have some ideas for how to do this and will cover them in Chapter 5.

CHALLENGING BEHAVIORS

Difficult behaviors, such as meltdowns, tantrums, aggression, and self-injury, are common in ASD although not part of the diagnostic criteria. These difficult behaviors are the natural outcomes of navigating the world when struggling with the constellation of behaviors that we've described so far. Regardless of the fact that these challenging behaviors are not considered part of the diagnostic criteria in ASD, they are still a big deal if you are a parent.

You will probably be interested in separating out such problems to address them. A 45-minute tantrum, rare in most children, will be all too familiar to many of you. Other challenging behaviors such as hitting or kicking others, or self-injurious behaviors like head banging or biting one's arm, are also rare or nonexistent in typically developing children yet all too common for many individuals with ASD. (See the box on the following page for more examples you may be familiar with.) These behaviors, whether driven by inability to engage in flexible thinking, sensory processing difficulty, or social information processing difficulty, then further disrupt coping, social relations, and flexible thinking— leading again to an unfortunate self-reinforcing cycle. Again, we'll talk later about what we are now learning about how to begin to address this.

Do Behavior Challenges Appear Mainly in Kids with Delayed Language or Intellectual Development?

We once thought the answer to this question was yes. But we now know that more is going on with behavior problems. There's some truth to the idea that problems are naturally worse when a child has fewer language or intellectual resources at her command. Yet recent studies have found varying associations: Some show that verbal abilities do not correlate with frequency of challenging behaviors at all. Others suggest that atypical sensory processing or rigid patterns of thinking are more likely to account for challenging behaviors than verbal or cognitive ability. Still others show that many verbal children with ASD who have age-appropriate cognitive abilities also demonstrate increased rates of challenging behaviors. Obviously what's behind challenging behaviors is complex.

Common Challenging Behaviors in ASD

Challenging behaviors, in and of themselves, are not part of the DSM-5 diagnostic criteria. But it's important for parents to recognize them as part of ASD so that they can be addressed appropriately, rather than viewed as unconnected willfulness or defiance—an attitude that can stand in the way of helping your child overcome the core challenges of being on the autism spectrum. Here are typical challenging behaviors you might see:

- Tantrums and meltdowns
- Noncompliance: refusal to comply with a demand or request
- Self-injurious behavior, such as hitting oneself, head banging, biting one's arm or finger
- Aggressive behavior, such as lashing out at another with hand or foot, biting, throwing objects, or breaking objects
- Elopement: running away and not returning
- Less common challenging behaviors, including:
  - Fecal digging and smearing: Digging refers to inserting a finger into the rectum, and smearing refers to smearing the feces on property or on oneself or others
  - Food refusal: refusing to eat anything
  - Pica: eating things that are not food, such as nails, dirt, paint chips, etc.
  - Rumination: spitting up partially digested food and rechewing it
  - Induced vomiting: purposefully vomiting

For a given child in a given situation, understanding what is driving the challenging behavior is critical to developing strategies for managing it. You essentially have to be a private investigator, digging for clues and putting together the pieces to solve the mystery. Fortunately, there are steps you can take to identify the root of the challenging behavior. Those steps are based in our understanding of learning principles discovered long ago by psychologist and philosopher B. F. Skinner. These behavioral principles, in fact, provide the basis for several empirically supported treatments for autism, treatments based on applied behavioral analysis, or ABA.

ABA as the Key to Figuring Out What's Behind Challenging Behavior

So, how does ABA work? In the world of behavioral psychology, any given behavior (which we'll label B) is preceded by something, an antecedent (which we'll call A), and followed by something, a consequence (C). (This sequence is often called A-B-C.) Behaviors are influenced by antecedents or consequences and can increase or decrease in response to changes in both. So, by determining the antecedents and consequences that influence a given challenging behavior, you can identify what you need to change to reduce that challenging behavior. Then you'll systematically change that antecedent or consequence, monitor the impact on the behavior, and if needed, revise the antecedent or consequence that you're changing until you see the behavior change.

Here is an example from my (Bernier's) clinic: Joe is an adolescent with ASD in a self-contained special education classroom. He is one of eight students who range in verbal ability and have a variety of special education needs. Joe's cognitive abilities are delayed, and he uses short sentences to communicate. He lashes out with his fists against his peers at least once a day at school, and these challenging behaviors are impacting the whole classroom. Using an A-B-C approach, we'll define our behavior of interest as Joe's lashing out with his fists. We start by exploring the antecedents. What happens before Joe lashes out? By asking some questions we see that the lashing out occurs at all times of the school day, but primarily during art class and music class, which occur at different times during different days of the week. The lashing out does not happen during structured academic time. Joe has no insight into why he lashes out. By doing some observing in the classroom we see that there are no assigned seats during art and music class, the level of sensory stimulation is much greater in those classes, and the students move freely throughout the space, while Joe remains relatively stationary once he enters his classrooms. We look closely at the consequences. What happens after Joe lashes out? Two things emerge. First, he gets some physical space from his peers, who shy away from him, and second, he spends some time in the reserved quiet space with his aide. Given the antecedents and consequences, one of our working hypotheses might be that the sensory stimulation is too much for Joe, and he is attempting to regulate how much sensory stimulation he gets. Lashing out is rewarded since it leads to a reduction in stimulation (the quiet space). So, we can then intervene by changing the antecedent. We can reduce the degree of sensory stimulation by changing the physical structure of Joe's space during class so that students don't bustle around him and find a location where the noise and visual stimulation is reduced. We might also teach him to tell us when he needs a "break" from the stimulating classroom, by teaching him to raise his hand rather than lashing out. By quickly removing him from the overstimulating situation when he raises his hand, we teach him that he doesn't need to lash out to cope with a difficult situation.

> Identifying what happens before and after a challenging behavior can help us modify it. That's the basis of ABA interventions.

We would want to track the frequency of the lashing out prior to intervening, conduct our manipulation of the antecedent, track the frequency after we intervene, and check that frequency to make sure the frequency of lashing out is reduced. If it is not, then we need to revise our hypothesis and consider a different intervention approach.

There are an endless number of possible antecedents or consequences that we can examine and manipulate to change behavior. However, you don't need to be Sherlock Holmes to figure it out; you just need to be willing to put on your detective's hat and give it a shot. And, in addition to your sleuthing and manipulating antecedents or consequences, training your child to develop coping skills can be critical to reducing challenging behaviors.

More recently, research suggests that children with ASD engage in fewer challenging behaviors when they learn and use better everyday coping abilities, such as requesting a break. This new research evidence suggests that self-regulation skills and application of adaptive coping abilities are the essential ingredients for managing challenging behaviors—and more critical than overall communicative ability.

> Recent research shows that it's not how well your child can communicate as much as his self-regulation skills and coping strategies that will help discourage challenging behaviors.

Self-Regulation

Self-regulation is the ability to effectively fine-tune our behavior, thinking, attention, and emotional experiences. This may include inhibiting an impulse or controlling an emotional outburst but can also mean staying on task or applying resources to a given task. Children with ASD have difficulties with many aspects of self-regulation. Thus, many children with ASD can be impulsive, easily distracted, fail to follow through on nonrewarding tasks, or display very challenging behaviors. Although well-designed studies have found that children with ASD do not differ from their peers in their body's emotional response to frustration—that is, both groups of children show increased physiological arousal to frustrating experiences—children with ASD use fewer goal-directed self-regulating strategies to defuse that frustration. The strategies tend to include verbal outbursts or meltdowns instead.

It's important to consider self-regulation and its relation to ASD from a developmental perspective, though. Young children struggle with self-regulation. This is part of the normal process of development. We don't bat an eye when a toddler flops down and cries when it's time to leave a fun birthday party because it's not atypical. And that makes sense. The part of the brain that helps us regulate our behavior, the prefrontal cortex, is still developing and learning to manage the signals that come from other parts of the brain—in this case parts of the brain that drive and monitor our body's emotional experience. Similarly, the parts of the brain that serve language are still developing, and we rely on those parts of the brain to label our body signals tied to emotion. So, with the thought of an end to the fun at the party, the toddler's brain signals a flood of activation in both the brain and body that underlie what we as parents would label sadness. However, the toddler doesn't yet have that cognitive label to put on the signals coming from his body and brain and doesn't yet have the ability to choose how to respond to those signals. Therefore, he ends up struggling to regulate the emotional flood coursing through his brain, and the result is flopping on the floor and crying.

For an individual with ASD, we know that development and functioning of the prefrontal cortex can be slower to develop. The prefrontal cortex is the part of the brain that helps us pause and reflect for a moment on cues we're getting from the environment or from within ourselves or to choose which behaviors are appropriate for a given situation. Further, as we've already discussed, language deficits are often common in ASD, as are difficulties with making sense of emotions. This brain circuitry underlying language and labeling of the body's emotional experience is tightly connected to regions of the prefrontal cortex, and so the atypical functioning of this circuitry means that your child with ASD will be acting more like a younger child.

So, when your 8-year-old with ASD has tantrums or flops on the floor or struggles to manage her emotions, this is likely a reflection of the fact that her prefrontal cortex is still develop-

> The prefrontal cortex helps us decide how to behave, and this part of the brain develops more slowly in children with ASD. So it's no surprise that your child with autism may have tantrums or display other challenging behaviors you would usually associate with a younger child.

ing. Even during toddlerhood, children with ASD are more likely than typical children to have difficulties in self-regulation. This highlights the fact that the delays in the development of the neural circuitry underlying self-regulation ability are already present. This familiar example of a toddler melting down when confronted with impending departure from a cake-filled birthday party highlights the importance of both the ability to identify and label one's emotional experience and the ability to select appropriate behaviors in response to that emotional experience. Given that these skills are challenging for children with ASD because their prefrontal cortex is less mature, it is understandable that your child will become more easily upset.

Is It Autism or Just Everyday Misbehavior?

One question that comes up in our respective clinics regularly is whether a particular behavior is part of autism or part of normal development or something else entirely. In most instances, challenging behaviors stem from delays in self-regulation related to a child's difficulties with identifying, understanding, and managing his emotions. Billy was a child diagnosed with autism. His mother described how sometimes Billy won't notice when other children in his kindergarten class are crying. As a volunteer in Billy's class she has had the opportunity to observe her son's behavior relative to his peers on the playground and in the classroom. She noted that he does not seem to even recognize if a child falls down, bumps her knee, and starts crying. Billy will just keep on playing and then become frustrated if his injured friend won't respond to him, even though she is crying. She said that similarly, in their home, he won't notice if she is ill or sad. She wondered if this was part of autism or just something about her son.

Billy's mom's observation is mirrored in scientific research conducted in the 1990s as scientists were trying to understand the social challenges young children with autism faced. In one study focused on emotion perception in children with autism, a scientist sat across the table from a toddler playing with a toy workbench, hammer, and nails. During the interaction, the scientist pretended to bang her finger with the toy hammer and proceeded to cry quietly and adopt a facial expression of distress for 30 seconds. This simple interaction was repeated with dozens of preschoolers with autism, toddlers with developmental delay, and toddlers with typical development. It was also repeated with the parent playing the role of the scientist. The interaction was recorded so that coders, unaware of which diagnostic group the children belonged to, could rate the amount of time children attended and responded to the scientist's or parent's distress. It turns out that the children with autism attended much more to the toys in this situation. They attended to the distressed actors far less than their peers did. This lack of attention to another's distress exemplifies the difficulties with processing the emotional experiences of others discussed earlier. So, in Billy's case, his lack of recognition or response when others are hurt or ill seems part and parcel of autism and reflects challenges with making sense of the emotional world.

Importantly, these difficulties with processing social information hamper learning about emotions and therefore understanding one's own emotional experience. One of our roles as parents is to help support our children's learning about the emotional world. We do that by putting labels on behaviors we observe in our children in particular contexts. To the toddler who screams no and cries when it's time to leave the birthday party, we might say, "Oh, you're so sad that you have to leave because you were having so much fun." We provide the label for the child to tag to the feeling in his body. Over time and repeated experiences, the associations can be made between the label and the feelings in the body and ultimately the situations in which those feelings arise. Well, as you can readily imagine, if you have a hard time recognizing other people's different emotional experiences and understanding what your own body cues are, it's difficult to know what to attach that label to. Add to that difficulties in processing language, and you've got challenges compounding other challenges. The result will be distress without the necessary tools to label it or choose a productive way to regulate or reduce it. The distress therefore looks from the outside like aggression and lashing out, tantrums and meltdowns, and self-injurious behaviors like head banging or finger biting.

In autism, a variety of situations can lead to distress. Difficulties with communication can lead to frustration. If you are stuck doing something that you really don't want to do and you can't let people know that, that is distressing. If you are in a situation where the sensory experience is overwhelming, as with loud noises or uncomfortable sensations, that is distressing. If you have gastrointestinal distress or haven't slept well or are having subtle seizure activity, that is horribly uncomfortable and distressing. Or, given difficulties with being flexible in your thinking, if you held expectations for how an event was going to unfold, but it didn't, you would feel distressed as well. All of this distress, without adequate tools for recognizing, labeling, and identifying the appropriate coping strategy to regulate it, is a recipe for challenging behavior.

Fortunately, children with autism can learn how to cope with a variety of situations, and many learn to navigate the world well without meltdowns. Again, in these situations, it can help to adopt the role of a private investigator so you can sort out why your child is upset. Further, by modeling coping skills, such as requesting a break for your child, you can begin to show her the tools she needs to be her own private investigator. Following that will be the important task of choosing the appropriate strategy to use to manage that distress. She can learn the A-B-Cs of behavior to identify the antecedents and consequences of her behavior, in this case her distress. Your child can begin to make associations between the labels you use when she has a meltdown when plans change and then learn what the appropriate coping strategies are for managing that distress.

The recent scientific advances in autism have outlined what the essence of autism is. At the core of this incredibly heterogeneous condition we see the importance of social motivation, the critical contribution of social information processing, the challenges of sensory processing, and the role of inflexible thinking in the behavior we call autism. That spectrum of challenges interacts with medical conditions and cognitive capabilities to drive the unique profile of behavior you see in your child. As a result, every child's autism is unique, and as we've hinted, and will discuss further in the next two chapters, this is driven by the many distinct causes of autism and the varied changes that occur in the brain in autism.

◈

Take-Home Points

- The basic characteristics that define autism are (1) impairments in social communication and interaction and (2) the presence of restricted and repetitive interests and behaviors.

- Understanding how these characteristics interact to hinder learning can help us turn things around and stimulate learning.

- Children with autism do not lack motivation overall; they lack motivation specifically for the social world. This can change if the social world is made more rewarding for them. There are strategies for doing so.

- Children with autism vary with respect to how rewarding they find the social world, from those who avoid the social world to those who very much want to be part of the social world but find it confusing and overwhelming.

- Every child with autism is different, but recent findings from genetic research show us how two seemingly different characteristics— such as sensory sensitivities and reduced social motivation—can both appear in children on the spectrum because they are caused by the same genetic mechanisms.

- MRI scans are helping us identify the areas of the brain that are different from the brains of typical children—and in turn are helping us design behavioral interventions that can shift those areas to "normal" in many children.

- Challenging behaviors are not part of the diagnostic criteria for ASD, but it's important to recognize them as part of ASD so that they can be addressed appropriately, rather than viewed as unconnected willfulness or defiance—an attitude that can stand in the way of helping the child overcome the core challenges of being on the autism spectrum.

• Understanding the triggers and consequences of challenging behavior can help parents and professionals identify what to change to reduce that challenging behavior.

3

WHAT CAUSES AUTISM?

One of the most common—and understandable—questions parents ask when their child receives a diagnosis of ASD is "What causes autism?" You may have already come across some claims; unfortunately, many are mere speculation, and some are explained in a way that ends up increasing confusion. To be fair, the complexity of what causes autism can make it a challenge to explain or grasp. In fact, over the last several years, scientists have discovered that autism is even more complex than we thought. Front and center here is the recognition now that ASD is an umbrella term that likely includes different conditions with different causes. In most cases, we can't determine the cause of autism for a particular child (except in a minority of cases, where a genetic mutation may be identified). What we do know based on the most recent science is that autism is caused by a mixture of rare genetic mutations in a subset of cases and a combination of common genetic susceptibility and environmental triggers in other (probably the majority) of cases.

You have probably heard arguments about "nature versus nurture." In fact the history of theories about autism is littered with arguments favoring one cause over the other. With our new understanding, we recognize that these either-or theories are false. An interplay between genes and environment is practically always involved.

A SHORT LOOK BACK: THE PAST CENTURY IN THREE PARAGRAPHS

Early theories of autism, in the 1940s and 1950s, basically asserted that children's problems could be traced to the early parent–child relationship. We know today this relationship is very important—in fact we harness its power to help treat children with ASD. But it's not the cause of autism. For example, one early idea was that children with autism were "turning inward" because they were not getting the love and attention they needed from their parents—especially their mothers. You can imagine how troubling this was to already frightened parents. This was a case of mistaking a correlation for a cause. After all, it does sometimes happen that a parent withdraws from a child with autism to protect against his or her own emotional pain. The parent responds this way because the child is unresponsive or difficult to read. In other words, the cause and effect are the opposite of what those early clinicians surmised.

Fortunately, the field moved on. By the 1960s a biological and genetic theory of autism was already gaining ground. A major turning point was the publication of a study of twins in 1977. In that landmark study scientists traveled throughout England identifying all twin pairs where at least one twin had autism—they found 21 pairs in all. They then simply looked at how often identical twins, who share almost 100% of their DNA, had autism, compared to fraternal twins, who share about 50% of their DNA. They reported that both identical twins had autism much more often than the fraternal twins. In fact, in that particular study, no twins in any of the fraternal twin pairs both had autism, but in 36% of the identical twin pairs, both twins did. Even with the tiny sample size (by today's standards), that result was impossible to reconcile with the "refrigerator mother" hypothesis and highlighted the role that genetics plays in the development of autism.

Subsequent twin studies that used newer diagnostic definitions of ASD and overcame some of the methodological limitations of that first study confirmed this picture, finding that in almost all identical twin pairs both twins had autism, further underscoring the strong genetic influence on ASD. Since that initial pioneering study, the genetic story has taken center stage—it has at times, perhaps, even been overemphasized, as by now we have also learned of many environmental influences on autism (although parenting does not appear to be among them). We'll detail those in a moment, but for now it's important to realize that parents don't cause autism, that genetics plays a strong part, and that early environmental insults also play a part. We'll break the genetic and environmental elements apart for simplicity and then bring them back together at the end.

GENETICS AND AUTISM

We mentioned twin studies; family studies also support a genetic element (even though families share both genes and environments). Based on current estimates, autism occurs in approximately 1 in 59 children in the United States, or about 1.5%. But if a family has a child with autism, the chances of the next child having autism increase to about 1 in 5—or about 20%. That's a fairly large increase—more than 10-fold. And if a family has two children with autism, the chances that the third child will have autism increases to about 1 in 3.

The field no longer relies on twin and family studies, however. The revolution in genetic research in the past decade has enabled us to focus on the genes directly in molecular and laboratory studies.

This is a complicated endeavor, however, precisely because autism is what is known as a "complex" disease. Unlike "simple" conditions like Huntington's disease, where a single genetic mutation is the cause, autism (like most other traits and conditions) is usually caused by a combination of factors, which can be different for different individuals. We now know that autism, like many other complex disorders, is associated with disruptions to specific single genes (although these are rare), with structural changes to the chromosomes that influence gene functioning, and with a combination of variations in multiple genes, as well as contributions from several specific environmental factors.

> About 1.5% of American children develop autism—a figure that increases to 20% when the family already has a child with autism and to about 33% when the family already has two.

Hundreds of autism-risk genes have been identified so far, and one educated guess is that 1,000 different genes and genetic events might play a measurable role in autism in the entire population. Some of these genes are very rare but, when present, are highly likely to result in autism—in those rare cases, we are fairly confident about what caused the child's autism. Other genes are common but play only a slight role in tipping the scales. (Also, certain rare mutations are associated with higher rates of certain medical conditions, such as seizures or gastrointestinal problems. It can be helpful to have this information so you can watch out for these conditions and ensure they are treated quickly.) That's why genetic testing is now recommended when a child has autism even though it is still rare to have a positive genetic test even if a child has autism.

The Latest Research into Different Types of Genetic Factors and the Risk of Autism

Because the genetic story has been developing so rapidly just in the last 5 years, it's worth your while to get a basic overview of the latest findings and understand where this work is likely to go. The five most-studied types of genetic factors that can increase the risk for autism are *de novo* single-gene mutations, *de novo* chromosomal changes, inherited mutations, "polygenic" effects, and an effect called mosaicism.

Single-Gene De Novo *Mutations*

Sometimes there is an unexpected change in a gene's code that prevents that gene from making the protein it is supposed to create. These mutations are how evolution works—by randomly trying different changes—but some of these mutations are harmful. Sometimes they disrupt proteins necessary for healthy brain development and therefore increase the risk for autism.

The surprising recent finding is that many of these single-gene changes are not inherited at all—that is, they are not in the DNA of the parents. Rather, autism seems to involve changes that arise anew either in a parent's egg or sperm at some point in the parent's life or in the baby at or shortly after conception. These are referred to as spontaneous or *de novo* mutations for that reason. These types of mutations actually occur in all humans and are usually harmless. But when they happen to affect a gene involved in brain development, they can increase the risk for autism or other developmental disorders.

Chromosomal De Novo Changes

The changes just mentioned alter the DNA sequence and impact a single gene. Sometimes, however, the genetic change is made in a portion of the chromosome rather than in a single gene. As a quick reminder, chromosomes are the structures located in the nucleus of each cell that contain long strands of information that provide the code for our genes. There are many genes located on each chromosome. We normally have 23 pairs of chromosomes, and each pair contains hundreds to thousands of genes. A small part of the chromosome can be missing or duplicated, and that disrupts the way genes located in that region operate. Some of these disruptions are inherited, as we'll discuss below, but again, in autism, many of these structural changes are not inherited; they are *de novo* as well.

Spontaneous changes to genes (those not passed down from parents) sometimes affect brain development and increase the risk for autism, so research is investigating why these mutations occur in the hope of discovering how to prevent them.

Here is an example of an early identified chromosomal change that we found in children with ASD that wasn't passed on from either parent. One of the most commonly associated genetic events in autism is a structural change to a particular area of the short arm of our 16th chromosome. These structural changes are called "copy number variants," and they include tiny deletions or duplications in the chromosome. In other words, the variants leave bits of DNA missing or bits of DNA replicated and inserted into the chromosome. In this particular region, there are nearly 30 genes. The chromosomal "hit" at this location therefore alters several genes, depending on the type of structural change. These changes are found in only 1% of all individuals diagnosed with autism. (And they can cause other conditions besides autism too.) One percent—so very rare. Most other genetic mutations are even rarer, found in only 1 in 500 children with autism, or fewer. That gives you a hint as to how rare each of these particular genetic events is and thus how difficult they can be to find—and to help you realize that while your doctor should order genetic testing just in case one of these is present in your child, odds are they will not be, even if your child has autism. Most cases of autism are due to either a mix of common variations of multiple genes (combined with environmental risks) or rare mutations to genes that we do not yet know are associated with autism.

Inherited Genetic Events

After reading about these *de novo* genetic changes you might ask, "Well, why does autism run in families?" It does run in 20–30% of families, and at times it's because single-gene disruptions or structural change to the chromosome are carried by parents without autism and then inherited by the child with autism. This adds to the complexity of the genetic causes of autism because it means that not all individuals with these genetic changes develop autism. This in fact is the most typical situation in autism.

> To complicate the genetic picture, not all children with spontaneous genetic changes develop autism—but whether they do often depends on whether they are boys or girls.

Furthermore, with some of these inherited single-gene variations, whether you have autism or not depends on whether you're a boy or a girl. That is, for some of these single genes that have been associated with autism, when a girl has that genetic change she will not have autism, but if a boy has the same genetic change he is more likely to have autism.

Let's return to the structural changes on that 16th chromosome. After first identifying changes to the 16th chromosome that were *de novo*, scientists started finding these disruptions in parents of children with these events. It turns out that these events did not always emerge only in the child with autism and were sometimes inherited from either parent.

Polygenic Effects: The Most Complex of All

It is likely that for many individuals with autism, the condition arises not from disruption to a specific gene or chromosomal region but rather from variation in several different genes. That is, in this "polygenic model," several genes affect a range of behaviors and abilities associated with autism, such as social motivation and ability to think flexibly. Variation to these genes results in a range of behaviors along these domains. The idea here is that autism is not an "all-or-none" condition. In fact, many of the traits associated with autism, such as sociability, flexibility, language skills, and attention, vary across the entire population. At the extreme end of these traits is the autism spectrum. Notably, some of these traits, such as exceptional memory, highly focused interests, and attention to detail, can be viewed as positive traits that, if applied correctly, are beneficial for humankind. This is why we also value neurodiversity and appreciate that while ASD has its challenges, there are many aspects of ASD that contribute to our society.

Mosaicism

Another source of complexity in the genetics of autism and a new theory about what might be contributing to the variability that we see in autism is the concept of mosaicism. Normally, every cell in the body has the same DNA—all that changes is how the DNA is expressed. But in mosaicism some cells within the body have a different DNA sequence because of copying errors that occur during cell division and replication. When those errors occur in development they can impact the degree of mosaicism. In autism, what current research is finding is that *de novo,* inherited, and other mutations we've discussed can occur in a mosaic fashion—and the extent of mosaicism may be crucial to whether the autism actually develops and how it appears. What this suggests is that the amount of mosaicism an individual has—how many cells contain these mutations—may prove key to autism appearance or severity.

Many Different Genetic Events = Different Causes in Different Children

In summary, we know at this point that there are many autism genes and genetic events; some are very rare, perhaps unique, and others are very common, meaning that they occur in the general population and therefore work in concert to increase the risk for autism. We don't yet know exactly what these genes do, but they probably influence the development of autism in different ways, even though some common themes are likely to emerge.

The natural conclusion, then, is that autism does not have the same underlying cause in each child—rather, there are subgroups with different causes. This in turn leads us to the idea that no single medical treatment or intervention is going to be appropriate for all children with autism and therefore we need to be more precise in our interventions. At the same time, we know that there may very well be some common biological pathways that will tie the different influences together, the way different streams converge on a river—so that many children may benefit from a given intervention even though the cause of their condition varies.

How We Try to Identify Common Biological Pathways

On the biological side, we are hoping to find that many of the seemingly different mutations ultimately have one or a handful of common biological pathways that affect the brain and contribute to autism, pointing the way to several types of interventions, each of which will work for many children.

Recently, one of us (Bernier) followed up on the earlier discovery that autism in some cases was associated with *de novo* disruptions to one particular gene. He and his colleagues wanted to find out whether children with disruptions to this gene had a particular form or type of autism. So, they took a second look at the subgroup of kids who had this particular rare mutation (see the details in the box on the facing page). It turned out that a particular profile did emerge. These children all had similar facial features: large head, prominent forehead, slightly wide-set eyes, and pointed chin. They all had autism but had a range of cognitive abilities. They all had gastrointestinal difficulties (marked by constipation), and many had significant sleep problems. This study marked the beginning of finding specific biologically defined groups within autism with clinical implications.

Looking for Common Biological Pathways

Scientists have studied dozens of genes associated with autism through this process:

An Example of Exploring Biological Pathways

Earlier research had shown that some cases of autism were associated with *de novo* disruptions to a gene called *CHD8*. *CHD8* encodes a protein called chromodomain-helicase-DNA-binding protein 8, which is essential for normal brain development. This gene was initially discovered by scanning through the DNA of children with autism, their parents, and unaffected children. I (Bernier) and my colleagues then followed up our identification of *CHD8* with more specific investigations. First, we obtained blood samples and, using special molecular techniques, scanned the DNA of thousands of children with autism and their unaffected parents, as well as thousands of other children without autism. We found the disruption to the *CHD8* gene only in children with autism (although only in a minority of them, 0.25% to be precise), and, strikingly, never in parents or in children without autism. So far so good. But we wanted to find out what this meant for the kids.

Next, we wanted to learn more about what this gene does. By scouring the research literature and reviewing what biologists had determined through many experiments, we found that this gene makes the protein early on in fetal development, in cells found in parts of the brain that have been implicated in autism—areas we discussed in Chapter 1—such as regions of the frontal cortex. Not surprisingly, though, the gene was also expressed in cells involved with how the body moves food through the gastrointestinal system. (It's quite common for a gene to perform different functions depending on where in the body it is placed, and for one gene to have multiple jobs.)

Perhaps most interesting to us, some of our collaborators made an animal model by disrupting this gene in zebrafish embryos and then observed the impact of this disruption in the animal. (Zebrafish are a good choice here because we can readily manipulate the genes of interest in this species, they develop quickly, and we can easily study their behaviors or physical structures.) Somewhat astonishingly, these zebrafish with disruptions to *CHD8* had very large heads and also had difficulties passing food through their gastrointestinal systems—reminiscent of the human children.

The *CHD8* gene codes for a protein that turns other genes on and off and affects the brain and other parts of the body. The genes that *CHD8* turns on and off have also been implicated in autism. You could think of *CHD8* as a master regulator switch that tells genes when to make their proteins and when to stop making them. It makes sense, then, that if this switch is disrupted other genes don't know when to turn on and off, and so proteins can fail to be made when they're needed or could fail to stop being made when they should stop.

1. Identify genes by finding disruptions to genes in large cohorts of individuals with ASD

2. Study individuals who have these gene disruptions

3. Examine how the genes work in the brain

4. Create animal models to test the disruptions' impact

The gene *SCN2A*, which has been associated with autism and has been studied in much the same manner as the *CHD8* gene described in the box, performs a very different function in the brain—coding for a protein that is embedded in cell walls and allows sodium ions to pass through them. This is really important because it's how neurons talk to each other—it's how the brain carries out day-to-day business.

Given the very different functions of just these two particular genes, it's easy to see that different approaches ultimately may be necessary to address the different sources of autism. And that is exactly what we predict will form the basis of "precision medicine" (a fancy term for individualized treatment) for autism in the future.

The exciting thing is that our understanding of the exact biological brain pathways involved in specific types of autism has led to ideas for medical treatments that could potentially correct those pathways. Thus far, we don't have any FDA-approved drugs that can correct any of the disrupted gene or brain pathways that cause autism. But such drugs are currently being tested in clinical trials; there is a real possibility of new drugs for at least a subset of kids with autism in the coming years based on these types of discoveries.

> *Learning more about the biological pathways that produce autism may eventually lead to the development of medications that can help at least some children with ASD.*

Another route to understanding the biological pathways involved in autism is studying a large population with the genetic change on the 16th chromosome described above. A team of scientists, including Bernier, conducted such a study. They created a welcoming website to let families know about the study and communicated to genetic counselors and genetic clinics all over the United States about it. Soon hundreds of families were interested in participating. The scientists conducted careful assessments of all the families, and it turned out that only about 23% of individuals with these structural changes had autism. Instead the children and adults had challenges ranging from language and speech disorders to intellectual disability to no observable medical or psychiatric problems at all. It quickly became clear that for this particular type of event, the presence of the structural change was not in and of itself sufficient to result in autism.

Essentially this means that although a few genetic changes appear to result in autism, most result in a variety of outcomes ranging from autism to other types of challenges to perhaps no challenges at all.

So, what is causing this puzzling variety of outcomes? Less is known about this, but the latest research is providing clues, and the clues point to multiple genes working together or the concept of mosaicism discussed above, as well as the phenomenon of epigenetics and the interaction between genes and risk factors in the environment.

> So far we know that a few genetic changes can result in autism—but sometimes the same changes result in other problems or no problems at all. Science is exploring the other pieces to this puzzle.

EPIGENETICS

Despite all the genetic progress, why do we still think autism is equally related to environments? To understand this and the full picture of autism, we need to review another critical concept: "epigenetics." Epigenetics means that experiences (or "environments") can create stable, enduring—yet potentially reversible—changes in gene expression. This is how the environment shapes development, traits, and autism. Ironically, or perhaps inevitably given how the body works, it does so by affecting the genes. This makes sense actually, since the body requires gene-built proteins and enzymes for every function, including brain operation. Gene expression refers to whether a gene is "turned on or off," that is, whether these proteins are made or not. These enduring changes in biology help us understand in a new way the importance of early life and ongoing stress, diet, exercise, and other influences.

A major driver of this evolving understanding is a field called "behavioral epigenetics." "Epigenetics" is a word with many meanings. Some people have used it simply to mean the vast array of developmental changes "on top of" the genome that occur during development. But here we intend a specific biological meaning. That meaning refers to specific stable biological changes in which the body forms a chemical marker to attach to the DNA molecule, changing its expression in a particular cell or type of cell. That change is sustained over time (e.g., during cell division). This definition is consistent with the current definition used by the U.S. National Institutes of Health.

There are different types of epigenetic changes, and each influences behavior and health. DNA methylation, the most common type of epigenetic change, occurs when a methyl molecule attaches to the DNA, in effect "turning off" the gene in that cell and changing the biological effects of the gene—including in the brain. Removing the methyl molecule can turn the gene back on. Some epigenetic

> *A lot of epigenetic change is caused by experiences, both biological and psychological, that "get under our skin" and are remembered in our biology.*

changes are preprogrammed in our DNA (like the differentiation of cells into neurons, skin cells, and so on during development). They can also be caused by random changes (just as genetic mutations can occur randomly). However, significant epigenetic change can also be caused by

---

Some Lifestyle Experiences That Can Lead to Epigenetic Change

- Diet and nutrition: what you eat
- Exposure to pollutants: what you are exposed to
- Sleep: when you sleep and how much you sleep
- Stress: physical and emotional stressors
- Exercise: when and how you exercise
- Learning and memory

experiences. In this way our experiences can literally "get under our skin" and be remembered in our biology. That is our focus here.

Therefore, whether a condition like ASD actually develops usually depends on two things: (1) our genes (our DNA) and (2) environmentally modulated gene expression or regulation. The gene regulation depends on numerous factors, including other DNA elsewhere in a person's genome, as well as different kinds of epigenetic effects, of which DNA methylation is one. Epigenetic changes like DNA methylation can be caused by both biological and psychological experiences, including nutrition, pollution exposure, stress, learning, and others. Several such lifestyle experiences are described in the box on the facing page.

Genotype × Environment Interaction (GxE)

At the level of biology, genes don't determine who you are; rather genes in interplay with the environment shape our development. In a statistical analysis, this interaction of DNA and experience is called "genotype × environment interaction," or GxE. You'll see a lot of studies on GxE if you venture into the medical or psychological literature these days. One way GxE carries out its effects is through epigenetic change. Epigenetic change is to DNA as control dials are to the electronic circuits on your car stereo. The stereo plays something very different when you change the bass–treble ratio, change the volume, or even change the station. After you change the settings, the new volume stays that way until you change the dial again. Yet the underlying electronics have not changed. Similarly, an epigenetic change happens on a gene in response to an event and then remains there, on the DNA, for a period of time until something happens to reverse it. The original epigenetic change may have been due to an event—say a very stressful pregnancy, or exposure to pesticides in the home, or lead in the school, or eating a very healthy or very unhealthy diet. The change then has a certain stability. Just like the radio volume doesn't change until something happens (you turn the dial again), the gene expression altered by the epigenetic mark after an experience may stay that way until another event reverses it or adds to it. For example, it appears that some epigenetic changes caused by stress can be reversed by aerobic exercise (see Chapter 6).

It is likely that most complex diseases and behaviors related to conditions like ASD are related to GxE. We call it GxE because the same epigenetic change doesn't happen to everyone who has a particular exposure or experience. The effect is an interplay between the experience and the person's other characteristics, including the individual's DNA.

To put it simply, complex diseases and disorders like ASD are rarely caused by genes on their own, but typically by specific sets of genes in the context of specific developmental experiences. These experiences act like triggers that bring to fruition the potential in the genes. What's inherited may often be a liability or vulnerability, rather than a full-blown condition.

> *What people inherit is often a vulnerability to a condition, and it is certain developmental experiences that actualize the potential.*

This makes sense if you reflect on it—when someone comes to work sick, not everyone gets sick even though everyone was exposed. Part of the reason is inevitably genetic differences in our propensity to catch colds. But on the other hand, the genetic propensity to catch a cold won't guarantee you catch a cold—if you avoid exposure, wash your hands, and are well nourished, you may avoid most colds even though you are genetically vulnerable. Vulnerability itself is a combination of genetic propensity, environmental risk and protection, and a particular disease-triggering exposure.

Some epigenetic changes are actually genetically driven—that's how cells become differentiated in development, for example (thus, brain cells or stomach cells have the same DNA—what's different is their epigenetics). Epigenetic changes can also happen because of random changes, just like we've seen with *de novo* genetic mutations. But our interest here is in the fact that significant epigenetic changes also happen through experiences during development.

The range of experiences that we now know can shape child development, brain, and behavior is impressive. It includes when a baby has a difficult birth, resulting in loss of oxygen to the brain (hypoxia), psychological stress on the parent or child, nutrition, pollution exposure, physical touch, and others.

It is here that we see the process by which genes depend on and interact with their environment during development. Epigenetics is biological proof that genes do not deterministically define people. Rather, at a biological level, genes always interact with the environment through epigenetic mechanisms. That dynamic interplay is what shapes our traits, including autism.

As a result, the story of epigenetics also has spurred new interest in how we might eventually identify new therapeutic agents and in the meantime how everyone can use the environment to help guide the growth and development of your child. Relevant to the theme of this book, in particular, then, is that we know that epigenetic changes, in some instances, can be reversed by new experiences that we can control, like exercise (Chapter 6).

For any given child, a unique combination of multiple genetic and environmental risk factors is likely at play. When the combination of those multiple factors reaches a threshold, autism becomes more likely.

> *Autism becomes more likely when a combination of many genetic and environmental factors reaches a threshold.*

ENVIRONMENTAL CONTRIBUTORS TO AUTISM

Quite a bit has been learned even in recent years about the most important experiences or environments that interact with our genetic background to influence the development of autism. Key environmental risk factors for ASD are often modifiable, which is great news because it leads to new ideas for how to prevent ASD or help children with ASD develop to their maximum potential. But it also points to the need to avoid overstating the power of the environment. As with most genes, as a general rule environmental risk factors influence the *probability* of developing autism but are not the only cause. And as with genes, these effects are not specific—most environmental insults, like most genetic markers, are also associated with other conditions or traits.

> *With disorders like autism we have to guard against exaggerating the power of the environment because those risk factors only influence the probability of developing the disorder and are not the only cause in any given case.*

The same picture actually holds for most modern illnesses, whether asthma, heart disease, or even cancer: we know there are genetic factors that increase somebody's risk, and environmental factors as well, but no single one provides a full explanation. What matters is the overall picture, and that's important to keep in mind—whether you're a parent or a research scientist or a clinician.

Factors That Come into Play before Conception and before Birth

Certain environmental factors increase the relative risk of having a child with autism. Again, however, risk factors influence the *probability* of developing autism but are not the only cause.

Here's an example that demonstrates a simplified way to think about this. As of the writing of this book, autism is diagnosed in a little over 1.5% of children (1.69% or 1 in 59) in the United States. Based on this prevalence estimate we can say roughly that the general chance of developing autism for any given child is about 1.5%. For children whose mother is obese during pregnancy, the risk (chance) of having autism is about 1.5 times higher. Therefore, this translates to about a 2.25% chance of having autism for a child whose mother was obese during pregnancy. Although there is a lot of statistical error in this type of example, it provides a way to think about the actual increased risk these factors confer in contrast to the large relative risk values.

The table on the facing page demonstrates the relative risk of several environmental risk factors associated with autism and the corresponding crude estimate of risk.

The vast majority of children born with these risk factors do not go on to develop autism (probably due to varying genetic vulnerability), but because the rate of each of these factors is higher in groups of children with autism, we consider it a risk factor—and potentially a clue to how autism develops, although we don't know if it is causal or if some unmeasured third factor explains the apparent association.

Older Parental Age

Scientists have long realized that parental age is associated with disorders that impact brain development, like ASD and intellectual disability, in two directions—when parents are very young or they are older than

Environmental risk factor	Relative risk	Actual risk estimate (based on current prevalence estimate)
Advanced paternal age	1.32	1.98%
Advanced maternal age	1.29	1.93%
Maternal obesity	1.47	2.2%
Pregestational diabetes	1.3	1.95%
Gestational diabetes	1.4	2.1%
Pregnancy interval < 12 months	1.9	2.85%
Prematurity (born under 36 weeks)	1.31	1.9%
Breech presentation	1.47	2.2%
Preeclampsia	1.5	2.25%
Fetal distress	1.4	2.1%
Induced labor	1.1	1.65%
Cesarean section	1.23	1.8%

average. In the case of autism and many other developmental conditions, older parental age is more heavily emphasized. A well-known example of older parental age increasing the likelihood of a condition is Down syndrome. The likelihood of a 20-year-old woman having a child with Down syndrome is about 1 in 2,000. That increases to about 1 in 30 when the mother is 45 years of age at the time the child is born. With autism the relationship between parental age is now clear as well—advanced parental age is associated with a 30–40% increased risk of autism overall. That means while the overall risk for autism is 1 in 59, or a little over 1.5%, for parents over the age of 35 the risk is about 2%. This holds for both the mother's and father's age.

Why does the risk increase with parental age? One route seems to be the *de novo* genetic mutations discussed earlier— they appear more likely as we age. Recall that these mutations can arise anew either

> Risk may increase with parental age because de novo genetic mutations appear to be more likely as we age.

in the sperm or egg cell (or shortly after conception). It turns out that *de novo* mutations are more likely to come from the segments of DNA passed down from the father—and are more likely the older a father is. This makes sense if we think about it. Millions of sperm are generated each day, and that means that there are a lot of opportunities for errors when copying DNA. So, it makes sense that if a *de novo* change is going to arise, it might happen during that sperm generation process.

Maternal Obesity and Diabetes

Maternal obesity and diabetes are other risk factors that we are realizing influence offspring brain development and risk for conditions like autism and others. While not showing the same strength of association between autism and parental age, several studies analyzed together have shown that both maternal obesity and gestational diabetes independently increase the risk for autism. The risk of developing autism is about 1.5 times greater (put another way, 50% higher) for a child with a mother who was obese during pregnancy than for a mother who had a normal body mass index. The risk of developing autism for a child whose mother had pregestational diabetes or gestational diabetes is 1.3 or 1.4 times higher, respectively, relative to a child whose mother did not have either form of diabetes. Once again, these effects are not going to definitely cause autism by themselves (most obese moms will still not have children with autism), but they combine with other factors to increase the chances of autism.

We are increasingly learning that fathers' health preconception also can influence child health and possibly autism risk. So, while we know more right now about mothers' health effects, we anticipate learning more about the role of fathers' health as well. Further, a great deal is being learned about epigenetic mechanisms that come into play related to mothers' and fathers' physiology and diet. Stay tuned for increasingly interesting, and perhaps hopeful, developments in this area.

Amount of Time between Pregnancies

Another prenatal consideration that has been identified as a risk factor is the time between pregnancies. A systematic 2016 review of several studies examining the time between pregnancies consistently found that intervals of under 12 months between pregnancies increase the risk for autism.

Medication during Pregnancy

Meta-analytic studies examining in utero exposure to certain types of medications have identified associations between medications and autism. The most well-established medication risk is for valproate. Valproate is used to treat epilepsy, as well as bipolar disorder and migraine headaches. A study in the United Kingdom found that women who took valproate or another medication to treat epilepsy while pregnant had children with higher rates of behaviors associated with autism. A large population-based study looked at all children born in Denmark over a 10-year period, comparing the number of children exposed to valproate in utero who ended up with autism and the number not exposed who ended up diagnosed. The data showed that children exposed to valproate were about four times as likely to receive a diagnosis of autism as those who were not exposed. The risk rate remained the same when the scientists accounted for parental age, gestational age, and a diagnosis of epilepsy for the mother.

Additional evidence that valproate is a risk factor for autism comes from animal studies. After being exposed to valproic acid in utero, mice showed social abnormalities and repetitive behaviors resembling some of the challenges observed in humans diagnosed with autism. Interestingly, recent research has shown that the offspring of the exposed mice end up with the same behavioral effects, highlighting the epigenetic effects of toxic exposures on our genetic background.

Selective serotonin reuptake inhibitors, or SSRIs (such as Prozac), have also been studied, because individuals with autism have altered levels of serotonin in their blood, leading to suspicions that taking SSRIs in pregnancy could contribute to autism. Based on several studies that have examined this relationship, however, scientists have concluded that the use of SSRIs during pregnancy does not appear to be causally related to an increased risk of ASD in children.

Folic Acid Supplementation May Be Protective—But Don't Overdo It

Pregnant women are appropriately advised to ingest sufficient amounts of folic acid, often by using supplements, because it prevents serious problems, in particular neural tube defects. Could it also protect against subtler effects like autism? While the study of folic acid supplementation in autism is still relatively limited, a systematic review of this literature revealed that when mothers supplement with folic acid during pregnancy, the risk for developing autism appears to decrease too. However, some studies and recent reviews introduce a critical caution: oversupplementation can *increase* risk. Further, even if you don't oversupplement, the benefit in relation to autism prevention may depend on the particular genotype or metabolic pattern of you and your child. So, while folic acid during pregnancy is certainly recommended, it requires careful medical consultation regarding total dosage across your diet and your supplements.

Early-Life Pollution Exposures

Chemical pollutants (called toxicants) are a major health risk—even a substantial contributor to mortality rates worldwide. This is why governments put some limits on use of these chemicals. Nonetheless, it remains clear from recent public health crises and news stories about lead and other toxicants in 2015, 2016, and 2017 in the United States and elsewhere that many public officials, school officials, and others are not aware of the relevant science. This fact, along with the sometimes alarming claims made in the media, convinced us it's important that you know where we actually stand with autism and chemical pollution.

First, we have to acknowledge the plausibility of the concern. The risk is not simply from an oil spill or special exposure—because exposure to "background" pollution is essentially universal on the planet now, we have to worry about supposedly "low-level" or "routine" pollution exposure. The risk to developing babies before and after birth from even this "background" level of toxicants is often underestimated, for two reasons:

1. Toxicant risk is often assessed in relation to physical health outcomes in adult animals, yet the developing child is more sensitive to toxicant exposures, even "small" exposures, than adults due to the child's faster metabolism.

2. The brain communicates with itself and grows through chemical signaling (hormones and neurotransmitters are, after all, trace

chemicals, and neural transmission also relies on trace metals), so the brain's development is exquisitely sensitive to chemical inputs. We now know the developing brain responds to toxicant chemical exposure at levels of exposure that do not cause physical illness or even physical symptoms.

The context is challenging for public health research. The chemical revolution of the 20th century has resulted in an explosion of chemical products that have entered children's environments. Over 80,000 chemicals are in commercial use. The *neurotoxic profile* (that is, how much they interfere with children's brain functioning) is unknown for nearly all of these. Fewer than 1,000 of these chemicals have well-characterized neurotoxic profiles, and even for those the effects on small children are often poorly studied.

However, we know that many of those that are well studied and have known neurotoxic effects even at low doses are common in the environment, so most children experience some exposure. These toxicants represent a policy headache for political leaders, a major challenge for business, and a significant worry for parents. Advocacy groups have sounded alarm bells and tried to get better regulation, but current public policies fail to provide adequate protections.

What toxicant chemicals are we talking about? In the case of autism, two main classes of polluting chemicals have been proposed as potential contributors in early life: heavy metals (especially lead and certain types of mercury) and organic pollutants (which might, for example, mimic hormones). The table on the following page provides a handy reference to the seemingly bewildering array of these chemicals.

Unfortunately, it's very difficult to keep our children entirely free from exposure to potentially neurotoxic chemicals. They get toxic chemicals into their bodies by mouthing toys and other objects, eating food with pesticides, drinking water with lead or other toxicants in it, breathing air pollution, and absorbing chemicals through their skin. The primary route depends on the particular pollutant involved. At the same time, the effect of these chemicals on children's development is notoriously difficult to study because we obviously can't do a gold-standard random-assignment experiment as we can with diet or exercise. The question parents ask most with such a complicated picture is "How worried

Examples of Known Neurotoxic Chemicals in Common Use

Pollutant	Association with child developmental problems
Metals	
Lead	Definite
Mercury	Definite
Cadmium	Likely
Manganese	Suspected
Organic pollutants	
PCBs	Definite
BPA	Likely
Organophosphate pesticides	Likely
PBBs	Likely
BHP	Suspected

should I be?" and in particular "What can I do?" We want to avoid alarm but maintain prudence, and we'll try to strike a balance here by hitting the highlights of what we know and a few basic recommendations for protecting your child.

In the case of ASD, many of these chemicals either have not been studied or have not shown any effect on ASD when studied. But there are some important exceptions. Recent scholarly reviews, while all noting the limited evidence and therefore differing on what chemicals or degree of risk should be emphasized, agree there is some role for environmental toxicants in the etiology of autism and that it is critical to study these toxicant exposures further. The timing of exposure may be very important—recent studies try to clarify when in pregnancy or when postpregnancy the most important effects occur. These appear to vary depending on the type of pollutant.

Particulate Matter in Air Pollution

Airborne pollutants are nonspecific—they include metals as well as particulate matter. But particulate matter is a special focus in the literature on ASD. While there has been some controversy, a comprehensive

2016 review of research studies confirmed that particulate air pollution increases the risk of autism. Those scientists examined all the studies that have measured parental exposure to particulate matter around conception and during pregnancy, as well as childhood exposure early in development, prior to receiving an autism diagnosis. The effects were quite clear. Importantly, these findings point not only to pregnancy, but also to the perinatal and early developmental periods following birth as potential risk periods for these exposures. A particularly careful review in 2015 helped clarify that controversy is coming from failure to differentiate the timing of exposure. In that study, the most potent risk for ASD in offspring was from pregnant moms' exposure to particulate pollution in the third trimester. This makes sense developmentally due to the rapid brain development happening for the baby in the last trimester.

Metals

A literature summary in 2017 found the following studies of metals and possible links to autism, with number of studies in parentheses: lead (25), aluminum (11), arsenic (6), beryllium (5), cadmium (17), chromium (11), manganese (14), and nickel (13). (It ignored mercury, which we discuss in a moment.) These exposures in the environment are potential threats to early development because they can disrupt brain growth and cell signaling in the brain in different ways. They do this in part through epigenetic signaling. One recent study demonstrated this by exposing rats to levels of lead similar to those most children are exposed to—levels that are statistically associated with neurodevelopmental problems in children. They found that the animals had altered behavior, and this was due to new epigenetic signals in their brains. Thus, again, we are not talking about special exposures like industrial accidents. Even low amounts, routine in our environment today, can affect child development. For metals, the primary effects appear to be from early postnatal exposure.

How potent a risk factor a particular toxicant is depends to an extent on whether the exposure occurs during a period of rapid brain development.

In the case of ASD, that review and others struggle due to wide variation in methodology, making it difficult to pool results across studies to get reliable estimates of population effects. That particular review concluded the best evidence of an association was for lead and cadmium. Other meta-analyses have also concluded lead exposure is associated with autism. However, it is possible this effect is modulated by the sex of the child (boys may be more sensitive). Lead's risk has hit the news again lately due to exposures in school water supplies. But it's important to realize that even though we've regulated lead in automobile fuel and paint, there is still plenty in our environment from all its prior uses (and current uses, like in some toys, airplane fuel, and the now infamous residential water lines). Almost all children in the world have measurable lead (as well as many other chemicals) in their bodies. One of us (Nigg) conducted a study of 300 children from the general population who had lead exposure that was average for the nation; 297 of them (99%) had detectable lead levels in their blood.

Mercury

Mercury is a metal, but a special case because its formulation, behavior, and action in the body are somewhat different from most other metals. Inorganic mercury exposures come from many current uses, including smokestack pollution from various industries as well as from the food chain (e.g., fish from polluted water). Note, however, that this is for inorganic mercury—that's different from the organomercury compound called thimerosal, used as a preservative in some vaccines—which turns out not to have a demonstrable association with ASD (we talk about vaccines in a moment). Organic mercury *is* associated with ASD and appears to have one of the most robust associations of any toxicant. The most detailed and comprehensive review and meta-analysis was conducted in 2017 and reported by Jafari and colleagues. They found that results depended on tissue studied (providing clues to metabolism as one issue for autism), but children with ASD had markedly higher levels in their red blood cells (more than double those of neurotypical children), as well as moderately increased levels in whole blood and in the few postmortem brain samples available. Interestingly, levels in hair and urine were no different than normal. This was interpreted as evidence that mercury plays an important role in autism, probably because children with ASD have abnormal detoxification and excretion of mercury. This is an important possibility and points the way to future enzyme and genetic studies to see if that is true.

Persistent Organic Pollutants and Pesticides

You've probably heard the most about this class of toxicants (e.g., bisphenol-A [BPA]), which are all listed in the table on page 78. While isolated studies have found associations of BPA and other organic pollutants with autism, that evidence has not yet accumulated to a decisive point. On the other hand, at least one major review this year concluded that evidence was growing convincing for pesticide exposures. The catch: these effects may be confined to relatively high exposures, not the general background exposure most children get. Nonetheless, taking steps to reduce needless exposure to bug sprays and related products is prudent while pregnant and while your child is young.

Complications at Delivery and Right After

Until now we've talked mostly about prenatal effects (with the exception of pollution exposures that can also be postnatal in affecting autism risk). Now we switch to effects right around delivery and after. Perinatal complications include events such as prematurity or infants born significantly later than the anticipated due date or complications associated with delivery, such as hypoxia (lack of oxygen), prolonged labor, cesarean section, and fetal distress.

In a recent study in 2017, scientists evaluated and systematically reviewed 17 studies examining the association between a comprehensive list of perinatal complications and autism. Combined, the studies included over 37,000 individuals with autism and nearly 13,000 comparison individuals. Perinatal factors for which a strong association with autism was identified included prematurity, breech presentation, preeclampsia, fetal distress, induced labor, and cesarean section.

From this review the relative risk for developing autism following each of these perinatal factors can be calculated. For example, the risk for children born prior to 36 weeks of gestational age is estimated to be 1.3, which suggests that these children have a 30% higher chance of developing autism. While that 30% number sounds large, this means that the risk rises from 1.5%, which is roughly the risk for the general population, to 1.8%. What has been observed in these studies included in the meta-analysis is that there are other perinatal factors that often co-occur with prematurity, suggesting that prematurity may actually be a marker of other perinatal complications. The relative risk for children with breech presentation was 1.47, a risk increase of 47%, which means an actual risk of approximately 2.2%. The relative risk associated with preeclampsia was 1.5, suggesting a 50% increase, and the relative risk associated with fetal distress is 1.4. Induced labor with medications such as Pitocin has also been associated significantly with an increased risk for autism with a relative risk of 1.1, or a 10% increased risk for those children exposed. Again, these effects are not specific; the risk of ADHD, for example, is also increased.

> While different perinatal factors slightly increase the risk of autism, we don't know whether the risk rises when a pregnant woman has more than one of these factors.

Does a Cesarean Section Increase the Risk of Autism?

This possibility has troubled many parents and caregivers. Once again, scientists recently (in 2014) conducted a study specifically focused only on cesarean section, in which they combined and reviewed 13 published studies relating it to autism. They found that children with autism were more likely to have been born by cesarean section than children who don't have autism. The pooled results suggested that the odds of developing autism following cesarean section were 1.23 times greater than the odds of developing autism born via vaginal delivery. That's a slight increase in risk. Like the other risk factors, the vast majority of children born via cesarean section do not go on to develop autism (probably due to varying genetic vulnerability), but because the rate of cesarean section is higher in groups of children with autism, we consider it a risk factor—and potentially a clue to how autism develops, although we don't know if it is causal or if some unmeasured third factor explains the apparent association. It is important to note that that small increased risk for autism has to be considered in the context of any other risks associated with that pregnancy and delivery. That is, the risk of death or other significant injury associated with not conducting a cesarean section may be very high in a given situation and justify the slight increase in risk for autism in the baby.

Other Perinatal Complications

Other perinatal complications do not appear to be associated with autism risk. These include vacuum extraction during delivery, vaginal birth following a previous cesarean section, anesthesia during delivery, physical trauma during birth, and a variety of placental disruptions (e.g., placenta previa, placental infarcts). Artificial reproductive technology has also not been associated with autism through meta-analytic study.

Is Inflammation or Immune Function a Shared Pathway?

Immune Function

A critical mechanism that may tie many of the environmental (and possibly genetic) risk factors together is inflammation and immune system function. Nearly all of the environmental risk factors we've discussed increase systemic inflammation, among other effects, and that in turn can disrupt brain health. For example, there is substantial linkage between inflammation response and both environmental toxicants and obesity. These inflammation responses in turn are typically related to epigenetic changes. Further, without regard to environmental risks, substantial immune system challenges have been linked to autism. For example, infections during pregnancy (which trigger immune activity and inflammation in the mother that spreads to the fetus) appear to elevate the risk for autism in the offspring. As another example, autoimmune disease (such as hypothyroidism) is correlated with autism. While the inflammation response to diet or toxicants may not be as strong as it is in response to infection, it may still be sufficient to account for the link between several early "insults" or "stressors" and a child's risk of autism. We therefore highlight the primary inflammation evidence a bit further.

The association of maternal infection with autism risk was established in a systematic review published in 2016 looking at 15 large studies that included over 40,000 children with autism. The risk is most pronounced for mothers requiring hospitalization because of the infection (suggesting more serious inflammation is related to a greater chance of developing autism). Further, the risk appears to depend on the type, timing, and site of infection. Different types of infections result in different immune responses, suggesting that the type of immune response may be a contributing factor.

> *Infections in a pregnant woman are associated with higher risk of autism.*

In addition to studying people, scientists have used animals to study how immune disruption and associated inflammation influence behavior. This is done by experimentally manipulating maternal immune activation in pregnant rodents, comparing them to rodents not challenged in that way, and then observing behavior in the pup offspring. These studies suggest that the pups show elevated social difficulties and repetitive behaviors. While it is obviously difficult to generalize from social behavior in rodents to social behavior in humans, we know that some of the biochemical bases of social behavior are shared across species. Thus these behaviors are thought to be reminiscent of human children's autism symptoms. So even though rodent behavior is only a distant counterpart to human behavior, the demonstration that complex behaviors like social interactions can be influenced by in utero inflammation exposures in animals supports the general possibility that inflammation contributes to autism.

Adding to the scientific evidence that disruption to the immune system during pregnancy is a risk factor for autism is the observation that a family history of autoimmune disease has been linked to autism. One review focusing on this line of research suggests that children whose mothers have a history of autoimmune disorders, including rheumatoid arthritis and celiac disease, are at increased risk for developing autism. Like all the environmental risk factors we've discussed already, when these factors occur in a mother, they increase risk but do not mean that the child will develop autism. What is driving that association? More research is needed to better understand this relationship. It could be that common genetic liability underlies both autism and autoimmune disorders, or in the case of rheumatoid arthritis it is possible that there is some prenatal antibody exposure or altered fetal environment that results from the maternal disorder.

Other Exposures

Vaccines

Vaccination controversy continues to make headlines as we write. The idea that early-childhood vaccines, such as the mumps, measles, and rubella (MMR) vaccine, are associated with autism has been tested in many ways. This is probably one of the most contentious and controversial topics we have in relation to causes of autism. We'll try to sort this out here.

First, a recent (2017) analysis of all studies testing the link between autism and vaccines using many methods concluded that *there is no association between vaccines and autism.* This means that if there is a signal there, it's too faint for scientific surveys to detect. Therefore, it's safe to conclude that for the vast majority of individuals, vaccines do not cause autism. However, we can't exclude the possibility that in rare cases a child had an underlying genetic or other medical condition (perhaps unknown) and that an immunization triggered the onset of the symptoms of that underlying condition. In this situation, immunization might have played a contributory role but was not solely the cause. If that type of event happened, but very rarely, then it would not be detectable in a population study. Certainly, given passionate anecdotal claims on this point, it's difficult to rule this out. At the same time, because autism onset and vaccine exposure often occur at the same time, an "illusory correlation" can appear even if there is no causal connection.

What is a good balanced conclusion on this difficult topic? Parents must weigh risks versus benefits of any medical treatment, whether for themselves or their child. However, one way to think about it is that the benefits of vaccination in preventing harmful diseases such as measles (not just for one's own child but for everyone in the community) are proven. Against that, the apparently very small risk of an adverse effect of a vaccination, in the vast majority of cases, argues for vaccinating children. In other words, if there are rare complications related to autism but we don't know why, then the probability of your child experiencing serious illness or death from disease if she does not get a vaccine is greater than the faint (even if more publicized) risk of an autism-related reaction. Overall, we advise you to maintain a regular vaccination schedule for your child.

WHAT SHOULD YOU DO WITH THIS INFORMATION?

Several practical steps are suggested by all of this information. We take the common questions and guidelines in order.

Should You Get Genetic Testing for Your Child with Autism?

By now many of you are wondering if you should get genetic testing for your child. The answer is "Yes!" In fact, genetic testing is now standard for children with autism, as outlined by the guidelines from the American Academy of Pediatrics. While for most of you the genetic test will not turn anything up or, even if it does, will not affect the plan of care for your child, the test will gradually help doctors learn more about autism and in a few cases may affect clinical care—and more genes will be identified each year. There's a scientific value too. For many genes, family groups have formed to connect families and also to link families with scientists who are focused on understanding how the gene functions and how treatments can address the gene's disruption. Finally, there's a chance that if you have a positive genetic test, you may be eligible for future clinic trials specific to that gene and your child.

Should You Get Genetic Counseling If You Have a Child with Autism and Are Pregnant?

Genetic counseling can provide helpful information for expectant parents, but given the state of science in the genetics of autism, the information will consist primarily of estimated risks for most parents. Those estimates can be summarized this way: In the general population, having a child with autism increases the risk of a second child having autism from about 1.5% to about 20%. Even if you have had genetic testing for your child with autism and a *de novo* genetic event has been found, the risk for having a second child with ASD remains at that population-based risk of approximately 20%. However, if a genetic event has been found for your child and it was inherited from either Mom or Dad, then the risk of having that event passed on to your second child is 50%. That doesn't mean your second child will necessarily develop ASD, only that the genetic event may be passed on. As mentioned, genetic disruptions do not necessarily mean that autism will develop.

How Can You Avoid Environmental Exposures and How Much Should You Worry?

For many of these environmental risk factors and others that have been studied by scientists, we now know there is in fact an effect on autism, though sometimes it is fairly small at the overall average level. However, these factors are very often highly related and occur at the same time for the same child. So, we suspect that the combination of multiple pregnancy-related conditions is what increases risk. Therefore, reducing any of them may be helpful. How can you do this? If you are a mom struggling with obesity, realize you have plenty of company. The many diets in our culture don't help. Some evidence suggests that extra omega-3 (fish oil) supplementation during pregnancy can counteract risks from obesity. Other studies suggest that total fat intake is the culprit, as well as that the amount of weight gained during pregnancy may affect risk. So work with your doctor on optimal weight gain relative to your starting body weight and body mass index, discuss the value of extra dietary supplementation, and modify your diet to a healthy level of fat with medical consultation. These steps should reduce risk. Finally, we know that stress is also inflammatory—if the shared pathway of all these risks is inflammation, then reducing stress during pregnancy will partially protect against these risks being amplified. Doing the best you can on these precautions is likely to be helpful. And realize that these contributions are only probable—most cases of autism can't be traced to a specific cause at this point.

Reducing stress during pregnancy where possible can prevent the inflammation that is a risk factor for autism.

The insight that we've gained into the causes and risks for developing autism have moved us forward considerably. These gains have put to rest troubling early theories about parents' roles in their child's development of autism. We now can see that some combination of specific or general genetic liability combined with a range of environmental nudges likely move children into the range of autism risk during pregnancy and in early life. These gains have provided insight into the mechanism that determines autism risk at the genetic and brain level, which has allowed scientists and clinicians to begin working on novel approaches designed specifically around an individual's biology. And these insights have provided us with information that guide the steps we can take to mitigate that risk.

◈

Take-Home Points

- *If you are planning to get pregnant:*
  - Be sure to take the recommended prenatal vitamins, starting before you plan to conceive.
  - If possible, space your pregnancies by at least 12 months.
  - If you are taking a medication associated with risk for autism, such as antidepressants, discuss your options with your doctor.
- *If you are pregnant:*
  - Seek prenatal care.
  - Get proper nutrition (including monitoring appropriate fat ratio) and rest.
  - Discuss omega-3 supplementation and folic acid dosage with your doctor. Reduce fat intake if necessary with medical consultation.
  - Plan your optimal route of weight gain with your care provider.
  - Engage in activities that reduce stress levels, such as exercise, yoga, and meditation.
  - Reduce toxicant exposures—minimize freshwater fish intake, keep your home dusted, consider testing your water or installing an effective water filter, consider spending the extra money to eat only organic fruits and vegetables. (See tips in Chapter 7.)
  - Avoid cigarettes, alcohol, and recreational drugs.
- *If you have a baby:*
  - Have your child vaccinated against serious childhood diseases; if you have concerns about vaccination, discuss these with your child's pediatrician, but we recommend going ahead with vaccination.
  - Be alert for ways to reduce pollution exposures—water, house dust, food. If you live in an area with high levels of air pollution, such as near a freeway, consider ways to improve air quality in your home with air filters.

- *If your child is diagnosed with autism:*
  - Ask your doctor to order genetic testing for your child. If your child has an identifiable genetic condition, ask your doctor whether there are any associated medical conditions, such as GI problems, to watch for.
  - Consider joining an online network of parents whose children also have that genetic condition.

4

HOW DOES THE BRAIN DEVELOP DIFFERENTLY IN AUTISM?

As we discussed in Chapter 1, autism is a developmental disorder. That means something is different in the brain and how it develops. Several brain regions and circuits have been found to develop differently in those with autism. Because there is wide individual variation, these brain measures cannot yet help us make diagnoses, but they do help us understand both the challenges and the strengths that are characteristics of autism.

A major insight in the last few years is that brain development is very dynamic, changing rapidly over time in response to different types of experiences. Scientists use the term "neuroplasticity" to refer to how dramatically the brain changes itself to adjust to development and to its experiences. It does so to a much greater extent than previously believed. We can use this knowledge to help us provide experiences, such as interventions, that will help shape the course of brain and behavioral development of children with autism, now and throughout their lives. Let's start with what we know about the brain in autism.

THE BRAIN IN AUTISM

Over the past three decades, scientists have conducted thousands of studies that paint a complex picture of structural and functional brain differences in individuals with autism. Careful systematic reviews of these studies reveal early emerging differences in the size, shape, and organization of the brain; differences in connections between brain regions; and different functioning of brain regions associated with social communication, social information processing, executive functioning, and repetitive behaviors—such as the amygdala and prefrontal cortex, which we discussed in Chapter 2.

Differences in Brain Structure

A systematic review published in 2017 of 52 brain imaging studies conducted since 2000 gives us one good summary. These were all studies that used MRI, a powerful, relatively noninvasive (if you call lying still in a tube noninvasive) imaging approach that provides a good representation of the internal anatomy and the connections between and within parts of the brain, in both size and apparent activity. Here are the major findings about the development of brain structure that emerged from the review:

- An association between autism and *a larger volume of cells in the cortex,* especially frontal and temporal regions. As introduced in Chapter 2, the cortex is the part of the brain associated with how we think, make decisions, and coordinate our actions. The frontal lobes specifically are involved in our working memory, ability to inhibit our actions, and motor planning, while the temporal lobes are involved in processing of emotions, language, learning, and memory, including interpreting social signals (such as facial expressions). The larger volume may seem counterintuitive—shouldn't it mean kids have better skills in these areas? However, it appears that this larger volume contributes to inefficient functioning in these areas. During development, the brain overextends its growth to allow for new learning, then gradually prunes unneeded or ineffective connections. Failure of this pruning can lead to a larger but less efficient and less adaptable brain.

- *Unusual variation in the thickness of the cortex.* That is, when measuring from inside to outside, the thickness of the brain is atypical in autism. This is a different structural brain measure, but it's similar to the idea of cellular volume and also consistent with the idea of insufficient pruning and the resultant less efficient brain.

  • *Alterations in the cerebellum,* a brain structure associated with balance and motor coordination as well as cognitive functioning. Alterations to this structure can impact the development of motor skills, learning, and cognitive abilities.

  • *Decreased overall size but increased volume within particular regions of the corpus callosum,* a structure that links both sides of the brain. Linkages between brain regions allow for efficient communication between brain circuits, so atypical linkages can result in delayed and problematic brain communication.

  • *Alterations in development of the amygdala,* a structure associated with emotional learning.

  • *Alterations in development of the hippocampus,* which is involved in learning and memory.

  • *Alterations in development of the basal ganglia,* which is involved in controlling physical motions. Alterations in the development of all three of these structures suggests that emotional learning, memory, and motor abilities may be disrupted.

What do all these differences signify? We're working on that, but the structural differences seen across studies do give us some direction on which brain regions are worth investigating. Also, these brain regions are all connected in circuits. It may be that only a small number of key circuits are involved in autism, but that the circuits involve several regions, so knowing which regions are affected may help us zero in on the relevant circuits.

> A recent research review showed us which regions in the brain are altered in autism and therefore where to target future research.

Functional Differences in Regions with Structural Differences

We also know that the regions that show structural differences function differently in autism. A key finding is that there is reduced activity in brain circuits during tasks that involve social awareness and understanding. Two significant examples:

• In groups of children with autism, the nucleus accumbens, a structure associated with motivation and reward, is less active when responding to social rewards, such as praise and smiling, than to nonsocial rewards, like money. In typically developing children brain activation is at least as high for social signals as for monetary signals. While we don't know the direction of effect for sure (do kids with autism have less brain activation because they are less interested in social cues, or do they have less interest in social cues because they have less brain activation?), these findings do fit with the general idea of less efficient processing of a particular kind of information in autism.

• Another example is the superior temporal sulcus, or STS (it is so heavily discussed among scientists that it has its own acronym). As discussed in Chapter 3, in most kids, the STS becomes active when a child is viewing biological movements, but in kids with autism, the STS does not respond as vigorously to nonverbal or implicit signals such as gestures, faces, and tone. Again, we can use this type of result to help us understand the challenge and struggles of your child. If she is not getting this information clearly in her mind, then of course it will be difficult for her to respond the way the rest of us do. It makes sense to link these brain findings with behaviors you are seeing in your child such as difficulty navigating social encounters, understanding another's perspective, and using eye contact and gestures to communicate because it helps us understand that these challenges are not willful or malevolent. These social challenges are based in differences in the way the brain processes information.

> *Brain regions that "light up" when a typical child is exposed to signals like facial expressions and body language are less active in children with ASD, which means those on the spectrum often have unusual social responses because they just aren't getting as much information from nonverbal communication.*

Differences in Networks and Connections

The circuits that connect brain regions may be where the real action is. Another major review in 2017 concluded that autism is associated with weaker organization among brain regions. Specifically, what we see is that the connections *between* the frontal lobe and the parietal lobe, which is toward the upper back of the brain, show less organization than the connections between regions *within* the frontal lobe. These weaker long-range connections between regions relate to deficits in social ability because processing social information requires rapid, efficient processing of information in disparate parts of the brain. The logic is that if those brain regions responsible for processing social information are not well connected, it will be difficult to make sense of the social world.

Imagine the array of wires behind your desk linking your computer, printer, mouse, keyboard, modem, external drive, and every other part of computer systems nowadays. They can be organized in an efficient manner, making it easy to clean, modify, add or remove components, and keeping signals running smoothly and efficiently. Or those connections can be disorganized, running in various directions and increasing the likelihood of problems. In the case of autism, all those wires connecting the different machines are not organized efficiently.

Taking this further: Let's say I'm (Dawson) swimming at the beach and a person on the beach jumps up and stands, looks out at the ocean I am swimming in with an animated expression on her face, extends her arms with index finger pointed, and shouts "Look!" I need to consolidate that information rapidly from disparate parts of my brain that process that information—face perception circuits (her facial expression and gaze), body movement circuits (jumping up and pointing), language circuits (she's shouting a warning), where I am (the ocean), the context (the beach), what I am doing (executing an impressive somersault in the water)—and accurately decide what to do with it. Certain brain circuits need to quickly consolidate all this information before translating it effectively to different brain circuitry to help guide my behavior in response. In this simple example, if that information is not pulled together efficiently *between* distinct neural circuits, the action I choose can have disastrous consequences (I could be eaten by a shark while waving to those on the beach who I believe are applauding my swimming prowess).

Strengths and Brain Function

Interestingly, the differences we see in brain functioning of individuals with autism, such as hyperconnections *within* brain circuits, might also contribute to having strengths in skills that don't rely on the affected or connected regions. About 10% of all individuals with autism have remarkable splinter skills, or savant skills—skills that exceed the other abilities of the child and at times the general population. These strong connections within neural circuits might account for those skills. For example, the occipital lobe is specialized for visual processes. If regions within the occipital lobe are tightly connected, we might see strengths in skills that rely on visual processing. It turns out that we often do see visual strengths as enhanced skills in autism. An easy example of this harks back to the *Highlights* magazines of our youth, in which you are asked to identify hidden objects within a picture. Individuals with autism tend to be able to identify those figures hidden among the background more quickly and accurately than their typically developing peers. While it is unclear if hyperconnectivity of the visual brain circuitry accounts for these splinter skills, scientists are working hard to better understand the connection between brain connections and behavior in autism.

> Brain circuitry in ASD is like the nest of wires under your desk: weak, disorganized connections slow down transmissions (e.g., creating social communication struggles in ASD), while unusually strong connections within certain circuits create extra-acute signaling (producing the savant skills seen in about one-tenth of individuals on the spectrum).

Differences That Predict Later Symptoms

Recent pioneering research is producing data that indicate we may be able to see signs in brain structure and functioning that predict autism before any outward signs appear. For example, certain differences in the growth of the surface area of the brain from 6 to 12 months of age seem to predict the "overgrowth" in the brain that happens from 12 to 18 months of age. Variations in these growth patterns are associated with the social challenges we see in autism. A recent study suggested that functional connections between brain regions at 6 months of age may predict subsequent emergence of autism. It's too early to use these findings in diagnosing children, but they raise the tantalizing possibility that we could eventually identify infants who may go on to develop autism using a quick screening test and then use a brain scan to get more information. Those who test "positive" even though no symptoms have emerged could then get behaviorally based interventions that might potentially prevent the symptoms from ever emerging at all.

How Do These Differences Operate to Result in ASD?

All of these findings give us focused hypotheses about brain development in autism. Scientists now suggest four main theories about the mechanisms behind the development of autism: the social brain hypothesis, the connectivity theory, the social motivation hypothesis, and the neural excitability theory.

- According to the *social brain hypothesis,* disruption to the structures and regions responsible for processing social information accounts for the development of autism. The findings from the structural, functional, and connectivity studies provide support for this hypothesis.

- According to the *connectivity theory,* fundamental disruptions to connectivity leave skills intact in some domains but create challenges in completing more complex tasks that require integration of multiple brain regions. The structural and functional differences that are observed in particular regions, according to this theory, are downstream effects of these poor connections. The connectivity studies provide support for this theory.

- According to the *social motivation* hypothesis, autism results from an initial disruption in assigning relevance and reward to social stimuli, leaving these infants inattentive to their social world. Findings of structural and functional differences in parts of the brain associated with reward, such as regions of the basal ganglia, provide support for this perspective. As with the connectivity theory, the structural and functional differences that are observed in particular regions are downstream effects of limited experience attending to the social world (i.e., underuse).

- According to the *neural excitability* theory, those who develop autism have differences in the likelihood that brain cells will respond to input in regions associated with processing social information.

None of these theories explains all the data, but each one incorporates and explains many of the brain imaging findings. It may be that different mechanisms are involved for different children. Given the different causes of autism, it makes sense that one theory about the brain in autism is not going to apply to all individuals.

Differences May Not Be Destiny

At the beginning of this chapter we noted that we now know the brain is plastic—that brain development is dynamic, changing in response to a lot of different experiences. This means that, just as some experiences may disturb development in a way that produces autism features, others, including interventions, can offer the promise of positive changes in brain structure and function. We can see this potential with an understanding of how the brain develops.

> *The brain's plasticity makes it possible for interventions and other experiences to create positive changes in the brain of those with autism.*

THE DEVELOPMENT OF THE BRAIN

The brain is not built at birth—it develops dramatically and fast before birth occurs. Brain cells of different types are produced at an incredible rate in the first four and half months of pregnancy. At some points, the rate can reach 250,000 new brain cells each minute! By the time a baby is born, the brain contains 100 billion neurons, which is almost as many as it will ever have (remember the principle of overbuilding and then pruning for efficiency, the way a potter puts out more clay than needed and then removes the excess to achieve the desired shape).

Cell Migration and Differentiation

Shortly after cell birth (and still during pregnancy), cells begin to migrate and differentiate into different kinds of cells (this is one of the things achieved by epigenetic signals, discussed in Chapter 3, and is why every cell in our body has the same DNA despite having different functions). Some neurons will become large, top-heavy neurons designed to send signals quickly from motor regions in the brain to the rest of the body to control movement, while others will serve as waystations translating incoming information from our sensory system and relaying those signals to parts of the brain dedicated to processing that incoming information. Experiences and insults at this point in development therefore have particular effects different from experiences or insults at another point in development.

Cell Maturation

Cell maturation begins next and continues through adulthood. During the cell maturation stage, the cell structures that gather information from other cells, called dendrites, and the structures that project onto other cells, called axons, develop to facilitate communication between cells and circuits within the nervous system. Cell maturation is highly dependent on life experiences and their timing. For example, musicians who begin playing the violin earlier in life have greater numbers of dendrites, representing greater maturation, in those regions of the brain associated with finger movement, than musicians who begin during their teenage years or those who try to pick up an instrument later in life. Does that mean we can't learn how to play the violin? Of course not, but the brain cells underlying the ability to perform that task will not be as mature as if we had picked up that violin and bow as a 4-year-old. We know from animal studies that the brain is more responsive to experience during early life than later, and this is why as adults we are somewhat less adaptable and have a harder time learning new skills than children do.

Pruning

We already mentioned pruning as another crucial process. Synapses are the connections made between neurons. As cells differentiate and mature they begin making connections with other neurons, and they do so incredibly rapidly. The brain is laying the framework to be able to do things and is readying itself for experience to help shape how it does it. It is as if a city were being built in a day with a detailed communication network—first the houses are built (cells and neurons); then they are wired together for communication (electrical and phone grid). The brain does much more than a city does, but the analogy may help. But it's also as if whatever electrical or phone wires aren't used just melt away—saving energy and interference in the grid. This is like the brain; over the course of development those synapses—those connections—are maintained only when they are used. The rest are pruned back, leaving only the regularly used connections. This makes the brain "less noisy" and more efficient.

Some pruning occurs in all brains, such as the way our senses develop. A drastic example comes from experiments in the visual systems of animals, which show that there is significant growth of synapses within the visual circuitry of the brain early in development. But when light is experimentally stopped from reaching the brain after birth (such as by restricting the animal to darkness or preventing its eyes from opening), those synapses are pruned away and the remaining, strengthened synapses focus on other sensory stimuli, such as sound or touch.

Other pruning occurs specifically as a response to a person's experience, a prime example being face processing. Babies are attuned to seeking faces right from birth, and infants can recognize, for example, monkey faces as well as human faces—much better than older children and adults can. That ability diminishes at around 6 months of age, because the brain has learned that distinguishing monkey faces isn't important and prunes those synapses.

Similarly, at birth infants can discriminate all the phonemes (the simplest units of speech) of all languages on Earth; the brain has grown a synapse for all possible words. But by age 6 months children recognize only the ones they are exposed to and now will learn their native language more efficiently. Importantly, it's not simple exposure to the stimuli that keeps certain language-related synapses intact. *The speech sounds have to be accompanied by social interaction.* So, listening to a foreign language on the television in the background is not sufficient to maintain those synapses. The sounds have to be socially meaningful or salient to the developing brain to continue to activate those neural pathways and keep the synapses functioning. The brain is smart!

SHAPING THE BRAIN

These studies into cell maturation, synapse formation, and pruning point to the incredible power of experience in shaping the "plastic" human brain. Early experience for some behaviors is critical and timing is important, but we now know it's never too late. Even though it gets harder as we mature, we can, for example, learn new languages even in adulthood. *The brain is more plastic than we think throughout development and even through adulthood.* Not only can we keep learning throughout adulthood—and learning means that connections between neurons are becoming stronger, cells are becoming more mature, and unused paths are being pruned away—but scientific studies have shown the brain can reorganize to compensate for stroke, traumatic brain injury, and amputation to varying degrees. People with an amputated arm have reported experiencing sensations of touch coming from their hand that is no longer there. Likewise, scientists using functional magnetic resonance imaging (fMRI) have found that stroke victims compensate for their injury through changes in brain organization. When healthy adults move their fingers, we typically see activation in characteristic and well-known parts of the motor cortex linked to the hand. When a stroke victim who has lost use of a hand gets rehabilitation and regains use, brain scans show the finger movements are recruiting other parts of the brain. The brain has created an alternative circuit for the necessary new learning during rehabilitation.

This type of plasticity can apply to a wide range of skills, including social skills.

A third example of the brain's plasticity comes from taxi drivers. Taxi drivers develop strong spatial skills as they navigate through city streets to take their fares quickly from one location to another. Scientists imaged the brains of London taxi drivers and found they had significantly larger posterior regions of their hippocampus—a region important for spatial navigation. That growth was directly correlated to how long the drivers had been operating taxis. Differences in other brain structures were not observed. In other words, the brain grew the networks to adjust to, support, and enable the extensive learning those drivers had undergone. The structure of this part of the brain associated with navigation changed over time through experience and learning.

Given that science has shown us that learning alters the brain and that the brain can respond to experience, it makes perfect sense to conclude that treatment approaches that change behavior will also change the brain—the brain is not destiny, but rather in significant part a reflection of experience and can modify with new experience. *Thus, it is a mistake to think that your child with autism has an unchangeable, "hardwired" condition. The brain has a lot of "soft wires" that can modify with the right learning opportunity.*

Behavioral Interventions That Help with Autism

We think the brain's plasticity is the reason why behaviorally based interventions that improve social communication skills and decrease challenging or disruptive behaviors are effective for autism. We know that these interventions, collectively called applied behavioral analysis (ABA), work. (We'll discuss them in Chapter 5). The new science of autism has also shown that behaviorally based therapies actually can change brain function; see the box on the following page.

About a decade ago, one of us (Dawson), together with colleagues, conducted a randomized, controlled trial of a naturalistic, behaviorally based intervention called the Early Start Denver Model, or ESDM. In that study 48 toddlers with autism were comprehensively assessed and then randomly assigned to receive either 2 years of ESDM therapy administered in the home for approximately 25 hours a week or a comparison intervention. This comparison intervention involved evaluation, recommendations, and referrals to area behavioral interventions. Following the first year of intervention the children underwent another comprehensive evaluation to assess their cognitive and adaptive skills and autism symptoms and then received another evaluation following the second year.

After intervention, the children receiving the ESDM gained in

ABA: Behavioral Treatments That Take Advantage of Brain Plasticity

ABA stands for "applied behavioral analysis." Most empirically based treatments use the principles of ABA, even play-based interventions such as the Early Start Denver Model (ESDM). ABA principles include the rules that govern how learning takes place. For example, positive reinforcement is based on the principle that when a behavior is followed by a reward, it is more likely to be repeated. Similarly, when we withdraw a reward following a behavior, that behavior tends to extinguish, or fade away, over time. ABA therapies, therefore, are those therapies that use these principles to promote desired behaviors (like social interaction) and reduce problematic behaviors (like aggressive outbursts).

cognition, language, and adaptive ability and had less severe autism symptoms. In this first-ever comprehensive, randomized controlled trial of this behaviorally based intervention, we saw gains in the children's cognitive skills and ability to make their way in everyday situations like getting dressed, interacting with others, and communicating. This study provided a capstone to the repeated findings from the many smaller studies of behaviorally based interventions demonstrating their effectiveness.

This study also examined brain activity to see the effect of the behavioral intervention on the brain. It used electroencephalography, or EEG, to examine any intervention-related changes in the brain's functioning. While recording the brain's transient electrical activity through electrodes along the scalp (with the EEG), the researchers showed the children pictures of faces and commonly found toys and then conducted the same procedure with typically developing children. They compared brain activity in response to faces (bio-

> The benefits of behavioral interventions don't cease when the intervention is over. After receiving intensive treatment, children with ASD had brain scans showing the same brain activity while viewing social information as typical children.

logical signal) versus objects. They found increased brain activity (and faster responses to faces) in the typically developing children and the children with autism who received 2 years of ESDM therapy, compared to the children with autism who received the community-based intervention. That is, the brain activity of the children receiving ESDM was similar to that of the typically developing children when viewing social information. The brain's activity changed and became more typical, mirroring the positive changes in behavior gained through intensive intervention.

This effect of behavioral intervention on the brain has been observed using other types of imaging studies as well. Scientists conducted fMRI in a group of 10 preschool-age children with autism prior to and following completion of a 16-week behaviorally based intervention called pivotal response training (PRT). The children watched point-light displays of biological motion (a moving body) and scrambled point-light displays while in the MRI scanner. They then received 7 hours of PRT intervention each week for 16 weeks. After the intervention period, they viewed the same displays while in the MRI scanner. A comparison group of typically developing children also completed the fMRI paradigm as a measure of what the expected brain activation should look like. Children with ASD showed differing brain activation in response to the simulated biological motion initially, but following the intervention, the activation mirrored that of the typically developing comparison children.

While the study of behavioral intervention's impact on the brain is still relatively new, these pioneering studies in autism highlight the effectiveness of intervention in changing both behavior and the brain. *It is possible to change the way the brain functions through intervention.*

THE ADOLESCENT BRAIN

You'll note, though, that the pioneering studies we just mentioned were conducted on young children with autism. What does that mean as our children get older? The brain continues to develop through adolescence, but there are important changes that happen during this time that have implications for your child's development. In fact, adolescence is a unique period in terms of brain development.

Scientists long thought that most brain development was finished by age 5 or 6. New understanding of brain development shows that this is far from the case and that there are specific major changes that happen during adolescence. To understand adolescent brain development, we use a special term: myelogenesis. This crucial stage of brain development begins prenatally and continues on through adulthood.

Myelogenesis concerns the creation of myelin. Myelin is like a fiberoptic upgrade. It speeds up neural transmission—brain communication within and across circuits and networks. Faster, more efficient transmission of signals between cells translates to faster, more efficient information grasp and more accurate response.

Timing is crucial here. The brain does not myelinate evenly. Rather, in typical development different parts of the brain are myelinated at different points in development. And this difference in timing in different brain regions is what is critical to understanding adolescent behavior and has implications for your child with autism. The parts of the brain that are myelinated first are those parts of the brain associated with basic processes, such as those that regulate breathing, arousal, vision, hearing, the motor and sensory systems. The parts that myelinate last are those parts associated with executive functioning, such as our ability to inhibit behaviors and hold multiple ideas in working memory as well as complex social cognitive behaviors like empathy. So, this means the parts of the brain that develop faster are associated with motor and sensory functioning and those that develop later are associated with how we measure risk, control our behavior, or make sense of complex social ideas.

A clear example of the differential development of distinct brain structures and regions comes from research looking at risk-taking behavior in adolescents. Using brain images of typically developing individuals across childhood and adolescence, scientists looked at the myelinated areas in the brain and found striking differences. They found that parts of the brain associated with reward and emotions became myelinated in adolescence earlier than parts of the brain associated with controlling behavior and assessing risk, which reached maturation later. *This means that the brain will respond more strongly and more efficiently to rewarding, risky behaviors than to complex ideas about later consequences or other people's perspectives.* This does not mean of course that teens are unable to inhibit impulses, but it means that the more well-developed structures that involve processing of emotions and desires may at times gain the upper hand of the less mature structures that help us manage our behavior.

Many of these gains in myelination are happening during the teen years. But other changes occur as well during these years: changes to neurotransmitter systems, increases in hormones that can differentially impact brain systems, and additional pruning that reduces the number of connections between neurons and increases efficiency of communication between brain cells.

So, what does this understanding of the developmental changes to brain structure and function during adolescence really mean? There are a few things to consider for your child:

1. *Providing relatively safe opportunities for risk-taking behavior may be a highly effective approach to teaching new skills.* This makes sense given that the circuits of the brain responsible for emotions and reward mature faster than parts that help prevent impulsive behavior or judge whether something is risky. So activities such as rock climbing (using appropriate protective measures) or participation in a ropes course might satisfy the desire for risk and provide a venue to teach executive functioning skills, like planning and working memory, which can hasten the maturity of those circuits.

2. *Heightened plasticity in the brain during adolescence offers another open window to focus on the improvement of social skills through behavioral approaches taught in naturalistic settings like school, where so much of your child's complex social world is unfolding.* These efforts to teach new behaviors could offer greater returns on investment.

3. *We also need to be finely tuned to the child's experience of the teenage world and be aware of the fact that we see increased rates of depression and anxiety in our children with autism.* As we mentioned in Chapter 2, as our children gain new insight into the social world, they sometimes feel isolated, alone, and without the skills to manage the relationships of the teenage world. It makes sense that depression and anxiety could follow. Your job as a parent is to keep an eye out for this, understanding that depression and anxiety may be harder to identify in your child. Some children with autism don't have the speech skills to communicate; others may not have sufficient language to describe these types of feelings; still others may not have a wide range of emotions such that you could notice shifts. Similarly, some symptoms of anxiety can be masked in children with autism because of existing rituals, repetitive behaviors, or avoidance of situations. However, by keeping a lookout for changes in your child's sleep, eating habits, energy level, or attending to increased irritability or looking out for loss of interest in activities that your child previously enjoyed, you can catch signs of depression. Similarly, if you're finding that your child is avoiding situations that previously weren't avoided or you see an increase in repetitive or ritualistic behaviors, it may make sense to think about anxiety. Very effective interventions and supports for both depression and anxiety are available. If you start to see these symptoms emerge and are concerned, contact your child's physician and share your observations.

Finally—and most important—the latest research, as we'll describe in a moment, shows us that brain structure and function can change in response to intervention much later than we ever imagined. The brain is resilient, plastic, and highly responsive to the interventions and supports we put in place to help our children. And we can put these supports and interventions in place to make those changes to brain structure and function and, therefore, behavior throughout development.

Brain Plasticity throughout Life

A perfect example of the lifetime dynamism of the brain comes from a study of face perception in adults with autism, conducted by one of us (Dawson) and a fellow researcher (her student Susan Faja). They developed a computerized training program that instructed individuals on how to look at and remember objects, such as faces and houses. They randomly assigned adults with autism who had difficulties with face perception to undergo the training program with a focus on developing either face expertise or house expertise. The adults were then tested on how well they developed skills to recognize faces and then also underwent an EEG testing session in which they viewed pictures of faces and houses. After the computerized training program, the adults who learned face perception skills showed improvement on standardized measures of face memory, and the adults who developed expertise in houses showed improvement on measures of house memory. The training program clearly worked at the behavioral level. When examining the adults' EEG responses to looking at hundreds of pictures of faces and houses, it was only the adults who underwent the face training who showed changes in the brain's electrical activity when looking at pictures of faces.

The thousands of studies of the brain in autism show us that in autism there are structural and functional differences that begin to emerge very early in development, long before the challenges your child with autism has even appear. But they also tell us that we can alter that brain development to help your child develop the skills to be more successful in social interactions, in managing anxiety, in reducing those challenging behaviors, and in learning everyday skills. *And we can make a difference in these ways to individuals with ASD throughout life.*

◈

Take-Home Points

- The brain changes much more quickly in response to development and its experiences than we once thought. Knowing which changes occur when helps us understand where development can go awry in autism and also where and how we might prevent or improve symptoms.

- We don't know enough yet to use our understanding of brain development in autism to diagnose ASD, but recent advances do tell us where to focus future research. That is, as of today there is no brain scan that we can use to diagnose autism, but the hope is to have a tool like this in the future.

- Differences in the brain that predict autism show up before outward symptoms appear. Knowing this, we can imagine that a quick screening tool could identify the potential for autism in very young babies, who could then receive a brain scan, and when those results confirmed this vulnerability, behavioral interventions could be used immediately and might prevent symptoms from developing at all.

- Treatments such as ESDM and PRT, which use ABA techniques, are effective because they're based on how we learn. They help children with ASD reverse deficits in social skills and control narrow interests and repetitive behaviors that are interfering with their lives.

- Adolescence comes with rapid brain development, offering new opportunities for growth, particularly social growth in naturalistic settings like school.

5

WHAT ARE THE BEST PRACTICES FOR HELPING A CHILD WITH AUTISM?

Our current understanding of autism has led to specific tools for helping individuals with autism. Because there are several paths that can lead to positive outcomes for your child, it is likely that one of the paths will work for you. Finding the right path can be confusing, however. Some popularized "solutions" can slow you down instead of helping, or at best are not effective. New, untested, and potentially harmful paths are proposed seemingly every day. While the Internet provides empowerment through unparalleled access to information, it also introduces a lot of noise and misinformation. Our goal in this chapter is to guide you to treatments and services that have proven scientific evidence for their effectiveness.

Another goal of this chapter is to help you focus on how important it is that assessments of your child and the treatment plans based on them consistently focus on your child's individuality. Everything explained in Chapters 1–4 has underscored the fact that autism is not a one-size-fits-all condition. It's essential to your child's best outcome that your son or daughter be viewed and treated as someone with autism who also has unique characteristics that must be considered in treatment planning.

Adding to the challenges of finding the right path is the reality that the path forward is rarely easy. Even when your family is on a realistic and worthwhile path with a good chance of success, plenty of hard work is involved. Everyone experiences ups and downs and seeming setbacks. Not everyone you speak with will have the same idea about what the right path forward is. Progress can be painfully slow at times, while at other times it can be rapid and exhilarating.

There is a familiar metaphor in the world of developmental disabilities that goes like this. Having a child is a bit like planning and going on a journey. As you anticipate the journey, you think about where you want to go, plan each part of the journey, and anticipate with eagerness your final destination. Having a child with a developmental disability such as autism is akin to stepping off a plane at your planned destination and finding that you've landed somewhere else. It's unexpected, disorienting, confusing, and even scary and can leave many parents with a sense of profound loss, at least initially. All of your preparation doesn't quite apply to the current situation. This is doubly true when you consider the many different shapes that autism takes. You may feel even more at a loss when you realize that advice that applies to other children with autism might not be a perfect fit for your child. So with this chapter we hope to help you take advantage of your knowledge of autism as a spectrum including wide variation and find the niche where your own child can get the best possible help.

STEP 1: GETTING AN EVALUATION

For practically everyone, getting a pro in your corner is a necessary complement to your own efforts. A professional diagnostic evaluation should tell you whether your child does in fact have ASD but also what individual needs your particular child has. The recent science in autism has highlighted that because not all children with autism develop in the same way, it's also important to get updated evaluations periodically as your child grows and develops.

It wasn't until 2000 that a synthesized practice parameter group came together to define the red flags that indicate an evaluation is important and warranted. While they are no longer "new science," they reinforce what signs are important to pay attention to. If you're reading this book before having had a diagnostic evaluation for your child, or you're concerned about a second child, see the box on the following page.

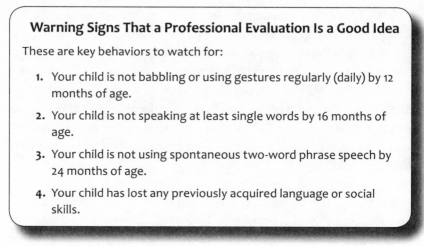

Warning Signs That a Professional Evaluation Is a Good Idea

These are key behaviors to watch for:

1. Your child is not babbling or using gestures regularly (daily) by 12 months of age.

2. Your child is not speaking at least single words by 16 months of age.

3. Your child is not using spontaneous two-word phrase speech by 24 months of age.

4. Your child has lost any previously acquired language or social skills.

As mentioned earlier, advances in autism research have not yet provided any biological diagnostic tests for autism. This means that there are still no genetic tests, blood assays, or brain scanning approaches that we can use to reliably diagnose autism. A diagnosis of autism is made based on expert observation in standardized testing situations, combined with careful history taking and interviews with parents. The following information will help you make sure you are getting the best evaluation science has to offer today.

How an Evaluation Can Lead to Individualized Treatment

To ensure that your child gets appropriate, and *individualized*, treatment, it's important to first determine that social difficulties with peers, limited eye contact, rituals, or struggles with transitioning from one activity to another exhibited by your child are actually due to autism rather than another disorder. A child with an anxiety disorder may not participate in social activities and can show particular ritualized behaviors to help reduce anxiety—but the treatment plan would be very different than it would be for autism. Similarly, a child with ADHD may have social difficulties following a pattern of failed friendships due to impulsive and dysregulated interactions—but need a different treatment plan than if she *also* had autism. Also, the picture can change with development, so it's wise to have your child reevaluated if new behavioral concerns arise.

After determining that your child's symptoms are best described with an autism diagnosis and not another diagnosis, determining the specific profile is critical so that an individualized treatment plan can be prepared. As we've emphasized, each child with autism is unique, and this variability across children with autism needs to be taken into account. There are no one-size-fits-all treatment plans. A good clinician will not simply say "Your child has autism; therefore we will choose this treatment plan." In fact, what is most important about the evaluation is understanding your child's unique strengths and weaknesses so that the care plan is specific to your child. As a result, a successful evaluation will not only determine the appropriate diagnostic label but also highlight the unique profile of strengths and weaknesses shown by your child.

> A fundamental aspect of individualizing your child's treatment plan is to incorporate the child's strengths and weaknesses.

How Do You Choose a Qualified Provider?

When a child's development needs to be assessed, it is of course always important to make sure the provider conducting that assessment is an appropriate fit in terms of training, credentialing, experience, and expertise. It may be even more important in autism that your provider have the appropriate training and education—such as that of a licensed psychologist, psychiatrist, neurologist, or developmental pediatrician—as well as enough experience to be up to date with recent advances in the field. Ideally, this means someone who specializes in autism, which means having had additional training or focused education specifically in autism and developmental disabilities, coupled with experience in working directly with individuals with autism. Last, ideally you want someone with expertise in the diagnostic process. You can ask some simple questions to ascertain how familiar and current with the diagnostic and treatment-planning process for autism a clinician is:

- "What experience do you have with autism?" You'll want to hear that the provider has had some recent autism-specific training and a currently active clinical practice within autism. By hearing about current trainings or active practice, you can be assured that your clinician is staying up to date with autism information.

- "What does your diagnostic evaluation process look like?" You'll want the provider to describe the process and hear that the provider uses the essential components of a good evaluation described below.

- "How do you stay current with your autism training?" You'll want to hear your provider discussing current research articles, review of the scientific literature, and attendance at conferences or continuing education classes focused on autism.

What Should You Expect during an Evaluation Today?

While there is some flexibility in how extensive the evaluation is, depending on your child's particular case, recent practice parameters and scientific consensus reports agree that the essential components of a good autism evaluation today include the following.

1. A review of the developmental history (your child's early social, communication, and behavioral development, medical and developmental milestone history). Recent scientific advances have highlighted the importance that early social deficits have for diagnostic specificity, so a thorough understanding of early social and communicative skills is critical.

2. Interview and ratings about current functioning, symptoms, strengths, and weaknesses. Sometimes questionnaires are used to gather information from a variety of people who know the child being evaluated. The recent development of several rating tools has aided in the rapid collection of important information about symptoms related to autism from multiple perspectives, which science indicates is critical to the diagnostic picture.

3. Direct observation of your child using commonly used autism diagnostic assessments.

4. Secondary or supplemental tests. These might include psychological testing to evaluate intellectual, language, cognitive, and

functional development or to examine co-occurring challenges such as sleep and gastrointestinal concerns or associated medical concerns (such as seizures). As we noted before, genetic testing is now standard even though it will be relevant to treatment only in relatively rare cases. Also be aware that there are assessments that are not clinically useful at this time, such as MRI scans for a child in the absence of seizures or other neurological signs.

It's common for each of these components of the evaluation to be provided by a specialist in that area (e.g., speech–language pathologist, geneticist, neurologist, gastroenterologist). Thus, the diagnostic evaluation often involves multiple providers with different expertise, so it is often referred to as an "interdisciplinary evaluation" (see the table below). This is perhaps one of the key advances in the evaluation of autism that has been driven by recent scientific findings. The critical contribution of GI problems to behavioral challenges, the rate of genetic disorders associated with autism, and the importance of recognizing seizures all

Common Providers Involved in the Evaluation and Treatment of a Child with Autism

Type of provider	Type of assessment
Pediatrician	Behavioral assessment, initial medical tests, including initial genetic screening
Psychologist	Behavioral and cognitive assessment
Psychiatrist	Assessment of psychiatric comorbidities, such as ADHD and anxiety, and the medications needed to treat them
Medical geneticist	Genetic testing, especially if specific genetic syndromes are involved
Neurologist	Epilepsy, seizure disorders, sleep difficulties
Gastroenterologist	GI problems
Speech–language pathologist	Speech delays, articulation difficulties, feeding problems, social use of language
Occupational therapist	Motor skills and coordination difficulties, functional play, sensory issues

highlight the importance of including other expert providers in the diagnostic process.

There are many ways to gather information about this history and current problems, and there are many ways to directly observe a child's behavior. To collect history and get an understanding of the current pattern of challenges, an interview with a caregiver or several caregivers is conducted by a clinician with expertise in autism. Sometimes this interview process happens with a single parent, and other times it can require interviews with multiple extended family members and include a teacher or two.

In recent years parents and others with intimate knowledge of children with autism have proven invaluable to increasing our scientific understanding of the condition. Parent and teacher reports help us identify patterns in children on the spectrum that we researchers can then study to gain understanding that produces information about cause and treatment. As a parent you are an expert in your child. You know when he is at his best and what supports he needs to navigate the day. You know how long this pattern of challenges has persisted, you know when there have been changes, and you can describe behaviors that may or may not happen during a short 45-minute interaction with a doctor and that could be missed during that direct observation of your child. Obviously such information is crucial to obtaining a complete picture of your child and her individual strengths, weaknesses, and needs.

> *Your expertise as a parent, and the collective expertise of other parents and teachers, is critical not only to designing the best treatment for individual children but also to increasing our scientific understanding of ASD by observing and describing patterns in children on the spectrum.*

Direct observation by the clinician is just as essential, because an expert clinician can capture symptoms or behaviors that will be missed in interviews alone. As discussed earlier in this book, clinicians today are not just trying to determine whether or not a child has autism, but also any qualifiers for that diagnosis that are relevant, any diagnoses in addition to autism that are contributing to the picture, and your child's observed strengths and weaknesses. The report resulting from the evaluation will outline what assessment tools and processes your provider used to make that diagnosis and specifically what the results of those approaches were to support the rationale for the diagnostic outcome. These assessment tools have evolved in recent years to help clinicians quickly and accurately diagnose autism. Prior to the development of standardized instruments like those listed in the box below, there was little consensus in diagnostic decision making, but these tools have allowed for greater standardization and far greater reliability in clinicians coming to the same conclusions about the same child. The report will then provide recommendations that build on your child's particular profile. It is these results and recommendations that will guide your decision making when putting together your family's care package.

Current and Commonly Used Diagnostic Tools for Autism

No one specific tool is effective by itself. The following are some of the common diagnostic tools that have strong scientific support.

- Autism Diagnostic Interview—Revised (ADI-R). The ADI-R is a semistructured caregiver interview. It is lengthy and not often used in clinical settings but is a powerful approach to gathering information systematically about children and adults with cognitive abilities over 18 months of age. Commonly used in research settings.

- Autism Diagnostic Observation Schedule, Second Edition (ADOS-2). The ADOS-2 is a semistructured observation (clinician–child interaction) that involves several interactive tasks. There are several modules based on language and age, each with different activities. The ADOS-2 takes 30–60 minutes to administer and requires expertise to administer and code accurately.

- Childhood Autism Rating Scale, Second Edition (CARS-2). The CARS-2 is a measure in which clinicians rate a child on the frequency, peculiarity, intensity, and duration of behaviors, such as communication, and social development based on their observations and information gathered during an evaluation.

- Gilliam Autism Rating Scale, Third Edition (GARS-3). The GARS-3 is a rating scale that can be completed by teachers, parents, or clinicians in about 10 minutes and assesses the frequency of autism-associated behaviors.

STEP 2: PUTTING TOGETHER YOUR TREATMENT PACKAGE

The careful evaluation process available to parents and children today is enormously beneficial in providing enough information to customize treatment for each individual child. But in all honesty, it presents challenges for parents. To do everything your child ideally needs as soon as possible could be a full-time job and often feels overwhelming. Most parents feel a great deal of stress as they try to absorb all of the new information they have received and put together a treatment plan that will be helpful for their child. And for most families, there's no getting around the fact that it's up to parents to put together and follow through on that treatment plan. A lot of support is available to you, but even accessing that can feel like another task for you to complete. Therefore in this section we'll tell you what we have observed clinically over the years that enables many parents to get the job done while keeping themselves and everyone else in the family sane and healthy.

If what we propose feels daunting, please keep in mind that we have scientific evidence that your persistence, advocacy, and attention will pay off for your child. The self-care that many shrug off as the hackneyed metaphor "Put on your own oxygen mask first" and place very low on their priority list has been shown to improve outcomes for the child on the spectrum and sustain parents for the years to come.

Here are some guidelines based on what we have seen work for family after family following an evaluation that indicates their child has ASD:

Ask Questions—Relentlessly If You Have To

It's the rare parent who goes through the evaluation process and leaves with clear "marching orders" in mind. Even after going over the diagnostic report in detail with your clinician during the diagnostic feedback appointment, the only thing you may remember hearing is the word "autism." Everything the clinician says after that could end up a blur in your memory. If this is true for you, you could reread the report the next day and realize you have questions—many questions.

So, begin by reviewing the report carefully and be sure to follow up with the clinician if you have any questions or disagree with any of the conclusions. It does not matter how minor you think the question may be. You want to understand every part of that report because you will be your child's key advocate and treatment coordinator. Don't hesitate to request a second feedback session so that you can get your questions answered face-to-face.

The report you received from your child's diagnostician will outline the key recommendations, or things you could do, to help your child and family. Making sure that you fully understand each treatment recommendation and why your clinician proposed it is important. This helps you consider what the priority is for that treatment component and if there are additional ways you can tweak or modify it, in conjunction with your child's clinician, to most benefit your child.

Organize Your Treatment Materials: This Is Not Busy Work

Getting organized at the start, even if you feel like you're still in shock and filled with questions about what the future will hold, will save you endless hassles later. Let's consider one family's experience. Joey's mother, Ellen, made copies of her child's report and shared it with every teacher and doctor her child came in contact with. She made sure she knew that report inside and out so she could speak to her child's strengths and challenges and could explain how the treatment recommendations built on those strengths and addressed the challenges. For her, and her child's caregivers, the report became extremely useful—because she had mastered what was in it. She put together a binder with a section dedicated to the paperwork associated with each particular part of the treatment package and color-coordinated it with the corresponding treatment recommendation in the report. She used that color-coordination system in the table of contents for her child's three-ring treatment binder. She called it her "three-ring-circus binder." For Ellen and for you, keeping the action going in all three rings requires prioritizing.

> Treating ASD over time is complicated. Don't be surprised if you need to keep track of lots of paperwork—possibly in what one parent called her "three-ring-circus binder."

Prioritize Recommendations and Tasks—You Can't Do It All at Once

One way to feel less overwhelmed, and to make sure what you do expend time and effort on is fruitful, is to prioritize each part of the treatment plan. Your clinician can help you do this. It's not possible to do everything at once, and it doesn't make sense to. Science has shown us that there are times when you need to tackle one piece before benefiting from the second. For example, when Molly came in with her parents, Richard and Diana, a key concern was that Molly struggled so much with disruptive behaviors that she was unable to attend or respond to the speech therapist. Science has repeatedly shown us that disruptive behavior can impede a child's ability to acquire new skills. In Molly's case, her parents and clinician decided that the highest priority was to address Molly's disruptive behavior so she could then work on developing social communication skills.

Ellen, Joey's mother, numbered each recommendation and prioritized with her clinician, because she knew she couldn't tackle everything at once. She highlighted parts of their report that she wanted to ensure everyone who worked with her child knew. And she identified key family members who could help her with different aspects of Joey's day, such as transportation to and from various appointments. This gave her some built-in time during the day for herself and other responsibilities.

Not everyone can be this organized, but Ellen's approach to organizing exemplifies the key pieces of a treatment package that fall to you as parent to the extent you can manage them: you must play the roles of organizer and ringmaster, armed with the information you need to advocate for your child, while making sure to take time for self-care.

Become Your Child's Treatment Coordinator—or Ringmaster

A key challenge is that your child is likely to be working with multiple agencies and people. Joey's evaluation led to recommendations involving his program at school, treatment approaches in the community, and components at the local autism center. The different agencies and providers didn't necessarily work together. Keeping the documentation and information about those different treatments organized was a challenge for Ellen, as for many parents. Yet it is also incredibly valuable if you can invest the effort to do so, because it helps you facilitate communication among all the people involved in your child's treatment. It can seem like a lot of work, yet that communication is critical. If all of the different providers are focused on the same goals, science tells us chances of success are magnified. Your clinical consultant can help establish consistent language (such as instructional terms or similarly defined goals) that everyone can use with your child to help solidify ideas across settings for her. Science shows us that this is particularly relevant for autism because of challenges that children with autism show in extending skills learned in one context to other contexts. Having goals that are being addressed in some capacity across settings, including home, will help your child generalize and solidify those skills.

Research also tells us that the simple act of contact between caregivers and providers on the treatment team on a regular basis improves outcomes.

Advocate for Your Child—It Makes a Difference

You've undoubtedly been advocating for your child since he was born, but now the scope of that function must expand. One of the most common concerns parents report to us is the constant struggle to access the treatments recommended for their child. And we have evidence from our years of clinical practice showing that serving as an effective advocate is key to realizing the potential for ASD treatment. It makes sense. Science shows that the children who receive intervention have improved outcomes, but it is the children whose parents advocate effectively who are able to access these services. Thus, those are the children with the better outcomes.

It all looks good on paper, but where do you find all these services? The wait lists are too long, or insurance won't cover the costs. Often, the school may be unable to provide the recommended resources. Advocacy for your child is the way. Here is an example:

Accommodations included in 12-year-old Tim's individualized education program (IEP) did not include some of the recommendations from his evaluation. Their provider explained to Tim's mother, LaTonya, that Tim had significant challenges with his slow processing speed, especially in making sense of what people said to him. So the recommendations for school included having teachers modify how they talked about his assignments, changing his seat to be less distracting, and shortening spoken instructions, yet none of these were part of the current IEP. LaTonya wasn't sure at first that it was worth fighting for these things, until she understood that her son's unique way of learning required this kind of support for him to succeed in school.

It's important to note here that it was LaTonya's understanding of what her son specifically needed and why that enabled her to advocate effectively for him. She was able to persuade the school to add these steps to the plan. This understanding also prompted her to find a new speech therapist to help the family learn to talk in ways that were easier for Tim to follow at home.

By really understanding your child's needs you can think creatively about how to meet those needs and be persuasive in communicating how those needs can be met. If the outcome of your child's evaluation indicated challenges in foundational social skills associated with his diagnosis of autism and the recommendation was for therapy based on applied behavioral analysis (ABA) because that is a key empirically supported treatment for your child's challenges, then you can use that knowledge to communicate with area providers, your child's school, your regional advocacy organization, your insurance company, or any other stakeholders.

> Advocating for your child with autism means being firm, persuasive, persistent, and polite. You're not being "demanding" when you request what your child needs and deserves, and trying to get it does not represent taking resources away from other children.

Be Persistent—It's Not the Same Thing as Being "Demanding"

Don't be reticent about calling your child's clinician back and asking for further explanation until you feel you really understand the rationale behind your child's treatment plan. And don't be afraid to keep asking for what your child needs. You will be empowered by the knowledge that your child needs and deserves this help. You are not trying to take away resources that other children need too. Simply state your case, politely and firmly.

Persistence is the most important part of being an effective advocate. Jill, the parent of 6-year-old Randy, is a member of an autism center advisory board. She shared with us that her one piece of advice to all parents is to be persistent. When Randy was 2, Jill and her husband, Jerry, had a gut feeling that something was not quite right with Randy's development but weren't sure what was going on. The pediatrician was also not sure but went ahead and put in a referral for an autism evaluation. They told Jill the wait for a diagnostic evaluation could be up to 9 months! Jill's persistent response was to call the clinic every single morning when it opened at 8:00 A.M. to ask if there were any cancellations that day. Her persistence paid off after 13 consecutive days of calling. There was a cancellation that day and she was able to take the spot. She was fortunate that she could take off work on short notice; obviously not everyone can, and this specific strategy won't work for everyone—but the idea is not to give up. You never know when a bit more persistence will pay off.

Take Care of Yourself—It *Can* Be Done

Many research studies highlight that the stress associated with parenting a child with autism outpaces the stress of parenting a child with other disabilities or chronic medical conditions. That stress can affect your marriage and your job performance and increase the chances that you will feel depressed and anxious. That is why, in your job as ringmaster, we want to highlight the importance of taking care of yourself. We realize that for most parents this falls to the bottom of the priority list. When Ellen says to her friend, "How can I take time for myself? I don't have enough time to manage all of Joey's appointments," she is speaking for many parents. Taking care of yourself is absolutely critical to being effective for your child, however. Self-care looks different for every person and is beyond the scope of this chapter, or even this book, to address fully, but it might include periodic respite care, an hour of massage each week, dedicated exercise time, or a grandparent or friend to lean on. See the box on the following page.

Self-Care and Stress Reduction

Scientifically Supported Methods to Reduce Stress

- Getting enough sleep
- Eating well
- Exercise
- Meditation and mindfulness
- Yoga
- Spiritual activities
- Spending time with friends
- Spending time with nature
- Reducing time looking at computer screens

Resources and Information about Stress Reduction

- *www.cdc.gov/violenceprevention/pub/coping_with_stress_tips.html.* The Centers for Disease Control and Prevention has a good summary of basic strategies to help you and your kids prevent or handle too much stress.

- *www.unmc.edu/wellness/_documents/FreeRelaxApps.pdf.* The University of Nebraska Medical Center has a nice list of relaxation apps that are freely available for download.

- *https://medlineplus.gov/stress.html.* Medline Plus, part of the U.S. National Library of Medicine, has a good resource regarding psychological stress with information, tips, resources, and links.

- *www.apa.org/helpcenter/stress/index.* The American Psychological Association has a comprehensive page outlining the impact of stress on the body and helpful tips on stress management.

- *https://healthfinder.gov/HealthTopics/Category/health-conditions-and-diseases/heart-health/manage-stress.* The U.S. Department of Health and Human Services website provides information regarding stress management approaches.

- *www.medicinenet.com/stress/article.htm.* WebMD's MedicineNet shares information regarding stress and stress management.

STEP 3: EVALUATING TREATMENTS

Your child's report will list a variety of recommendations that will include one or more treatments or interventions to build on your child's strengths and help address any weaknesses. This is great, because you can rely on your provider to help distill the thousands of reported autism treatments that are discussed on the Internet to what science suggests is appropriate. But it is still important for you to do your homework on the proposed treatments. Reading this book will help you get started on that homework. The most common types of interventions that will be recommended or considered as part of your treatment package include behaviorally based treatments; medication approaches; allied health services such as speech, physical therapy, and occupational therapy; school-based interventions; and interventions that fall under the category called complementary or alternative treatments. We'll equip you here to pick the best of these and evaluate the rest.

Behaviorally Based Treatments

Behaviorally based treatments are currently the only empirically based (i.e., science-based) treatments to address the "core" symptoms of autism—those challenges in social communication and repetitive/restricted behaviors. Behaviorally based treatments are those that rely on the principles of ABA. As noted in Chapter 4, these principles include the rules that govern how learning takes place. For example, positive reinforcement concerns the principle that when a behavior is followed by a reward, all other things being equal, it is more likely to be repeated. Similarly, when nothing rewarding follows a behavior, that behavior tends to fade away over time. Behavioral therapies use these simple learning principles to promote social communication abilities and reduce problematic behaviors, until eventually the new behaviors become automatic or natural for the child, to some extent anyway. The principles may be simple, and the treatment can really work—but the implementation takes great skill because you have to know what is motivating for a given child and what strategies will be most effective.

Further, it's challenging as a parent because many different variations of this idea are now marketed (and referred to by their inscrutable acronyms). Worse, some treatments claim to be behaviorally based but do not incorporate key aspects of behavioral principles and therefore lack scientific validity. The way through this is to basically ignore the name and find out what the exact elements of the therapists' plan are. But that said, a few well-known names are worth remembering. Here's what you want to see: The most well-studied and valid behaviorally based treatments for children during the toddler/preschool years (i.e., early intervention) are traditional ABA, such as discrete trial training (DTT), the Early Start Denver Model (ESDM), and pivotal response training (PRT). Autism Speaks (*www. autismspeaks.org*) is one resource that provides an updated catalog of information regarding the evidence supporting specific behaviorally based treatments. We list other resources at the back of the book.

> *If the name-brand treatments aren't available to your child, you can choose a program that has all the proven interventions' essential features.*

The Program Should Use Formal Measurement

But what if these "name" brands are not locally available? You can still evaluate the plan by looking at the components to ensure that the available program has ingredients similar to those in the proven treatments. The first such element is the use of formal measurement—the therapist should actually be using data collection and analysis to assess and monitor your child's progress. Ask to see these measurements. All evidence-based behavioral programs begin by developing a detailed treatment plan in which the therapist defines specific objectives or goals that the therapy should achieve. An example of such a goal is "When entering the therapy room, Johnny will look at the therapist and say 'Hi' 80% of the time." The treatment plan focuses on goals that the child should be able to achieve within a relatively short period of time. It is comprised of several objectives or goals across several domains (e.g., social, language, and toy play skills). After the therapy begins, the therapist collects daily data that monitors progress toward a goal, such as the frequency, intensity, and duration of a target behavior (e.g., eye contact). If progress is not being made, the therapist should modify the goal or change the strategy being used to achieve it. Ask how long a specific treatment strategy will be tried before it is modified based on the measurements. When skills are achieved, new goals are developed so that forward progress can be continuous.

The Program Should Be Based on an Individualized Assessment of Your Child's Skills

The second component is that the treatment plan should be based on an individualized assessment of the child's specific skills—that is, it should be tailored to your child's particular needs and developmental level. Beware of any treatment that is supposed to work for every child with autism and doesn't allow for individualization. To develop those goals and outcome metrics that are key to behaviorally based treatments, an individualized assessment of your child's abilities is necessary. For example, to achieve the goal of reducing tantrums, the therapist first measures the frequency, duration, and intensity of those tantrums. Measuring again later will prove whether or not they actually decreased. Similarly, to develop a treatment approach to reduce those tantrums, the therapist will need to identify the things that happen before the tantrum to precipitate them, called antecedents, and understand the consequences—the things that follow the tantrums and often reinforce and perpetuate the tantrums. All of this is explored as part of that individualized assessment.

The Goals Set Should Follow the Normal Developmental Sequence

Other components of effective behaviorally based interventions include a sensitivity to the normal developmental sequence. That is, we've learned a lot about child development over the years and understand the progression of key skills. For example, children learn to orient to the social world and other people before they learn to share attention with another person. When children learn to share attention with others, they can learn language most effectively. And so on. Incorporating this understanding of developmental sequences ensures that treatment goals aren't focused on skills that either require mastery of foundation skills first to become ingrained or would be learned much more efficiently if precursor skills were in place. Most empirically supported early behavioral interventions use a "curriculum" that describes a wide range of objectives across multiple domains (social, language, motor, toy play, and so on) according to developmental level. Following this curriculum ensures that behaviors are taught in a developmentally appropriate way that builds from one step to another.

A simple example concerns Meredith's son Michael, who was diagnosed shortly after the age of 24 months. Michael did not use any words to communicate at the time he was diagnosed. He also was not responsive when people called his name, and he rarely attended to people's faces. Before Michael's therapist focused on teaching him to use words, she taught him how to pay attention to others, use gestures, and engage in social interactions that would support the use of language. First she taught him to orient to his name and attend to the therapist and parent, then started in on teaching him the words for objects. You can make sure your therapist is considering the normal development sequence by simply asking him or her to provide a rationale for which goals are being targeted first. The therapist's response should reference the progression of goals building on one another.

The Therapy Should Be Enjoyable

Another critical component is that, for the most part, the therapy should be enjoyable for the child. There will likely be times when the child is resistant, especially when new goals are introduced, but a skilled therapist should be able to make therapy fun and engaging. The therapist should be sensitive to the unique needs and preferences of the child, such as becoming easily overwhelmed if the environment is too loud and stimulating.

The Program Should Gradually Move from a Therapeutic Environment to Environments in the Home and Community

The therapist should incorporate strategies that allow for the gradual, careful transition of learned skills from a highly supportive environment, such as a therapy room, to naturalistic environments, such as the home, classroom, and playground. This means that early on during behavioral treatment the therapist is going to include objectives that measure how well the child is able to "generalize" the learned skill to different situations, people, and environments. For example, the therapist should be asking you to use similar strategies at home and reporting back whether the child is able to use the skill learned in the therapy room at home. Be sure your therapist outlines a possible plan for generalizing learned skills to natural environments and with fewer supports. The idea is that over time that scaffolding will slowly be removed so that your child can practice and master those skills with fewer prompts, fewer cues, and more distractions.

As part of Michael's treatment program, he was consistently rewarded if he looked at his therapist's face when she called his name. During the first several trials, he received physical prompts to orient his face to hers, there were no distractions in the room, and he was immediately rewarded with tickles (in his case, his primary reinforcer or reward, which the therapist and parents discovered during the individualized behavioral assessment). Over several weeks (and many, many trials), the physical prompts were removed so that Michael was rewarded with tickles every time he made eye contact without that physical prompt guiding his face to hers. Then, as he mastered that, additional distractors were incorporated into the trial by calling his name when he was playing with a toy or engaged in another activity. The therapist then had him transition to other settings, such as his house, the park, and a store, and then increased the distractions in those settings by including other people. With each progression, the environment become more and more natural, so Michael was mastering use of his skills in the everyday world—it was getting more natural for him.

You Should Be Deeply Involved in the Program

Children spend most of their time at home, and every interaction at home is an opportunity for learning. Some therapies, such as ESDM, provide "how-to" books for parents where they can learn strategies to promote social interaction, language, and learning during everyday activities such as their mealtime, bathtime, or bedtime routines. Your therapist should allow you to be part of the therapy and coach you on how you can use similar strategies to achieve your child's goals at home. The therapist should also prioritize goals that are important to you and your family.

You should feel like you are not only part of the treatment team but also at the helm.

The Program Should Be Flexible in Other Ways to Meet Your Child's Needs

For many children with autism, behaviorally based therapies will be a key component of the treatment package. They are flexible so they can be adapted to what your child needs and your family can handle. The therapies can take place in the home, or at school; they can be skill focused or comprehensive; they can be of short duration or last multiple years; they can vary in intensity from an hour per week to 40 hours per week; and they can vary in their targeted outcomes, from language to behavior to everything in between. Whatever options you choose, if you ensure that the treatment contains the critical components highlighted in your child's evaluation and is geared toward the goals outlined for your child, the incorporation of behaviorally based treatments into your treatment package can be very effective.

Allied Health Profession Therapies

Speech–language therapy, occupational therapy, and physical therapy are also often recommended components of a treatment package for individuals with autism.

> *Other therapies can give your child the skills to get the most out of ABA and other ASD-specific interventions.*

Speech–Language Therapy

Given the core challenges in social communication inherent in autism, it makes sense for speech therapy to be a part of your child's treatment package. Speech–language therapists combine their understanding of verbal and nonverbal communication to help promote the development of skills in this domain for your child. Speech–language therapy can be conducted in a one-to-one scenario or in small groups or dyads. The benefit of small-group instruction is that your child is able to practice those social communication skills with a peer, which is where those skills are paramount. Speech therapists can also address other speech-related challenges your child with autism may have. Some children with autism struggle with articulation or the motor components of speech. This can affect the development of spoken language, as well as other oral motor behaviors involved in chewing and swallowing. Thus, many speech–language therapists will have expertise in addressing eating problems, such as gagging, picky eating, and others. A speech–language therapist can use specialized instruction to address these challenges, which can have a significant impact on the success of social communication. As you might imagine, when, thanks to the skills your child is being taught in therapy, other children can understand his speech, they will be more responsive and, as a result, reinforce the use of those skills. The result of that reinforcement is more practicing of those skills and ultimately a more successful outcome. Thus, addressing speech or language deficits becomes an important part of your treatment package.

Physical and Occupational Therapy

Relatedly, fine- and gross-motor challenges can impact your child's learning and development. Many children with autism have difficulties with gross-motor movements, such as being clumsy or not very coordinated, and also challenges with fine-motor skills, such as holding pens or using tools like scissors. Physical therapy and occupational therapy are well-supported treatment approaches to addressing these challenges. Improving gross-motor skills helps your child assimilate into the everyday activities at school or on the playground. Being unable to run, play tag, or jump in a bouncy house with her peers reduces her opportunities to engage with them, practice the key social skills she is working on in therapy, and ultimately develop the social competence that serves as the foundation for learning. You want to lower every barrier to her engaging with her peers and the social world. If she struggles with motor challenges, ensuring she has the appropriate motor skills, through physical or occupational therapy, can drastically increase her ability to engage with others.

Another domain of challenges that is often seen in autism is in sensory aversions or interests. Given the common occurrence of these sensory sensitivities, the presence of aversions or interests was added to the diagnostic criteria during the latest iteration of the *Diagnostic and Statistical*

Manual of Mental Disorders, or DSM-5. At times, these sensory sensitivities can become problematic. Randy, the son of super advocate Jill, had a taste sensitivity and licked everything he came in contact with, including other people he met. Marco, another child seen in my (Bernier's) clinic, was unable to tolerate not only loud noises, such as the school fire alarm, but also particular sounds like the hum of the lights in his classroom. He also struggled with tactile aversions, and had only a limited set of clothes he could wear, and lashed out when he was touched lightly on his skin. For Marco, occupational therapy was important to reduce his sensory aversions. His occupational therapist worked with him on wearing sound-reducing headphones and used a variety of exposures to train him to adjust to tactile sensations. Without that occupational therapy it would have been difficult for Marco to respond most efficiently to other aspects of his treatment package. For Marco's family the right path included not only addressing his social communication deficits using behaviorally based therapies, but also addressing his sensory sensitivities with occupational therapy.

WHAT YOU NEED TO KNOW ABOUT MEDICATIONS

No medications currently exist to address autism's core symptoms (although some new medications are in the pipeline). Systematic reviews and meta-analyses of clinical trials indicate that medications, however, can reduce some of the other challenges that your child faces, such as hyperactivity, aggression, or mood problems. Addressing these difficulties can help your child best benefit from autism-specific treatments.

Systematic reviews indicate that there are medications that are effective at reducing some of the challenging, disruptive behaviors we see in autism, such as self-injury and aggression. At times these behaviors can dramatically interfere with your child's learning other skills, so they need to be addressed immediately and directly. Medications such as risperidone and aripiprazole have been shown to be effective at reducing these behaviors. However, side effects such as weight gain and sleepiness are associated with the medications that are effective in reducing these behaviors. Thus, it is important that medication be used in conjunction with behaviorally based efforts and in consultation with a physician with expertise in autism.

Systematic reviews also show that medications can be helpful in reducing symptoms associated with depression, anxiety, and ADHD. Again, these medications are not addressing the symptoms of autism, but helping manage the symptoms of disorders that commonly occur with autism. Treating these associated disorders may be absolutely critical to improving outcomes for some individuals with autism and will help put you on the right path. Just as with medications taken to reduce challenging behaviors, the side effects of these drugs need to be considered, they need to be combined with other empirically supported treatments for these disorders, such as cognitive-behavioral therapy (CBT) or behavioral support, and a physician with expertise in autism will be an important ally on your path.

SCHOOL-BASED INTERVENTIONS

For most children with autism, school-based interventions will be a critical component of the treatment package. Your child spends many hours each day in school, and there are many opportunities to practice those key social communication skills that your child needs to master. The laws pertaining to education for your child and the tools and methods by which that education is delivered have been in place for many years, so what follows does not focus on new research or developments. Instead it represents, from years of work with families, our best advice on what to consider about your child's all-important school experience.

As with behavioral therapies, there are many terms and acronyms that can make finding the right path with your school confusing. Let's start with a critical one: IDEA.

IDEA stands for the Individuals with Disabilities Education Act, and it is the current incarnation of a law first passed in 1975, when educational services for children with autism and other disabilities changed dramatically. Prior to 1975, fewer than 25% of children with disabilities received education within public schools. Many families were directed to institutional settings, where the educational programming was limited and, in reality, mostly taught children with disabilities how to be successful in such settings. In 1975, Congress passed the Education for All Handicapped Children Act, mandating school services for children with disabilities. With this law, all children from birth to age 21 gained access to educational opportunities within the public school system with the directive that their educational needs must be met. While the federal law does not technically require states to participate, it provides incentives through funding when those states meet certain requirements. This 1975 law, also called Public Law 94-142, was renamed IDEA in 1990. Since that time the law has been amended several times to accommodate changes in state and federal laws, but the intent of the law has remained the same: to identify children whose disabilities interfere with their learning and provide a free and appropriate education (FAPE) in the least restrictive environment (LRE).

Let's touch on those two acronyms: FAPE and LRE. IDEA mandated free and appropriate education (FAPE) for children with disabilities. Free is pretty self-explanatory, but not surprisingly, one person's appropriate is not the same as another person's appropriate. The law defines "appropriate" as services that are adequate for a child to progress from grade to grade. It does not necessarily mean the best services possible. Many schools exceed adequate with flying colors, while other schools use approaches to meeting the adequate bar that fail miserably. Our years of experience working with families have shown that the quality can be highly varied even within school districts and dependent on the staff and administration. As you might imagine, this has become a source of frequent disputes between families and schools.

Another source of friction between parents and schools is the concept of the least restrictive environment (LRE). The focus here is on ensuring that children with disabilities are receiving education in the most normative settings, in classrooms with their typically developing peers, where the setting is appropriate for the child's learning. This is addressed with the following questions: Can the child receive an adequate education in the general classroom environment with additional supports? If a more restrictive setting is used, how can the child be integrated to the maximum extent possible and still receive adequate instruction? A key component here is that a child cannot be placed in an inappropriate setting just because it does not cost as much.

A key provision of IDEA is that states are obligated to identify and evaluate children with disabilities that require special educational services to ensure adequate education. This obligation pertains to all children, not just children within the public school system. This includes children who are at private schools, homeschooled, or homeless. After a child is identified, the local educational authority (LEA), which is the local school district, must then evaluate the child to determine if services under IDEA are warranted. This evaluation must be comprehensive enough to determine if the child's disability interferes with learning. A diagnosis in and of itself does not determine if special education services or supports are needed. The disability must interfere with the educational process. Importantly, educational progress is more than simply classroom learning. It includes classroom learning, but also learning in other settings such as physical education and transition services to employment, vocational school, or postsecondary education. Like your child's diagnostic evaluation, this school-based evaluation has a twofold purpose: (1) to determine if the child is entitled to services and (2) to identify strengths and weaknesses in order to develop the IEP.

The IEP provides the educational plan specific to your child and identifies educational goals, metrics for defining those goals and progress toward achieving them, and the services and supports that will be provided to meet those goals. Similar to other interventions, as our scientific understanding of the power of behavioral supports has increased, the incorporation of specific measurable, behaviorally defined goals has become increasingly sophisticated in today's IEPs. The IEP is developed by a team that includes the parents, teachers, other school officials, and the child. Other school officials could include a school psychologist, school social worker, or member of the administration. Others can also be part of the team, including providers working with the child outside of school, such as a behavioral therapist or psychologist. The team works together to develop goals that must be measurable, clearly defined, and tied to the outcome of the evaluation. All of the accommodations, services, and supports need to be outlined in the IEP document, the quantity and duration for each service need to be explicitly specified. Clearly outlining each of the goals, metrics, and supports makes it possible for progress to be measured and ensures that everyone on the team understands what will be provided. It will be critical for you to review the IEP document thoroughly to make sure you understand each component and are satisfied with the plan.

IDEA stipulates that special education services begin at 3 years of age but also provides programming up until 3 years of age. These early services are called Birth to Three early-intervention services. Like the variability in services for educational programming after age 3, there is a great deal of variability in these birth-to-three programs. Despite that variability the intent is to enhance the development of children with disabilities and increase parental competence to meet their children's needs. Also, similar to special education programming, after identification and evaluation, an individualized plan is developed. In this case, the plan is called the Individualized Family Service Plan, or IFSP.

Even if your child does not qualify for services under IDEA, there are other supports that can be put in place under additional federal laws. For example, the Americans with Disabilities Act and Section 504 of the Rehabilitation Act of 1973 both prohibit discrimination based on disability and stipulate that everyone must have equal access to services. So, if it is determined your child with autism does not need special services to progress from grade to grade but needs other modifications to access his education, then these laws may provide access to supports such as modified academic curriculum, seating in a particular location in the classroom, or leaving the classroom later to avoid crowds.

A critical message here is that you can and should be an integral part of your child's educational programming. Through active involvement in the development of the IEP, which can include bringing any relevant testing reports from other evaluators or providers to share with the team, you can ensure that the school plan is meeting your child's needs. Additionally, by maintaining active and direct communication with the school you can ensure that progress is being made, that changes to the IEP are being made when needed, and that the school and other members of your child's treatment team are working together. Finally, there are processes in place to ensure that your child's interests are at the forefront. These include your required consent to an IEP evaluation, the school's notice requirements, which ensure that all changes to an IEP must be provided in writing to the parents, specific mediation resources or due process hearings to facilitate problem resolution between members of the IEP team, and allowance for outside evaluations to be included in IEP preparation.

COMPLEMENTARY AND ALTERNATIVE TREATMENTS

Further complicating your task as treatment coordinator and advocate for your child, you will hear about various alternative treatments for autism and undoubtedly wonder whether they are worth including in your child's treatment plan. Describing each treatment in detail would fill up several books. So here we will stick to giving you some guidelines for evaluating these treatments as you encounter them. You should of course also consult your child's treatment team and pay attention to the research evidence as it becomes available.

What Is "Alternative"?

Many people in the United States use health care approaches that are outside of what is considered "standard medical care." These are referred to as complementary and alternative medicine (CAM) treatments. That is, they are complementary to the established interventions, to be used in addition to or in a supporting role, or they are alternative interventions to be used instead of established interventions. They are so widely used that the National Institutes of Health even has an agency that focuses on them: the National Center for Complementary and Integrative Health (NCCIH). Another term that is used to describe these interventions is "integrative medicine." Many well-established medical schools now have a division of integrative medicine that offers treatments such as meditation, dietary supplements, and other treatments that are not part of mainstream medical care.

Empirical support for CAM treatments ranges from relatively strong, such as the use of meditation to reduce stress, to nonexistent. Similarly, the treatments can range from relatively inexpensive and benign to extremely expensive and very harmful. Some treatments are relatively new, so the scientific evidence is lacking, whereas others have been well researched and are known to be ineffective.

An example could be the use of melatonin as an effective tool to improve sleep for children with autism. For many years this supplement was considered a CAM treatment, but it has now entered the mainstream, with systematic reviews of many trials indicating that it is effective as an approach to improve sleep for autism. As such, melatonin has moved from the nonestablished treatment category to one that is appropriately prescribed to children with autism in some circumstances. *(Caution: although it's over-the-counter, melatonin is a hormone, with particular risk for small children and teens—use with medical consultation.)*

Principles for Considering New Treatments

When you hear of a new treatment, your thoughts about whether it should be part of your child's treatment plan can be informed by these questions.

Does the Treatment Seem to Make Sense?

This is sometimes a tricky question to answer, so it is a great one to take to your doctor or your child's diagnostician. To get at the answer you might ask:

- "What does the treatment do?"
- "Do the proponents of the treatment base the approach on a theoretical rationale and if so, does the theory make sense?"
- "How does the treatment address my child's autism symptoms?"
- "Whom is the treatment designed to help and whom does it not work for?" No treatment works for everyone. Any treatment that supposedly works for everyone should immediately arouse your suspicion.

If the answer to the first question is that the treatment does not seem to make any sense, then you can move along and not include it as part of your treatment package. If, however, at least at first blush, it seems to make sense, there are a few additional questions to consider.

Is the Treatment Effective?

Effectiveness can be hard to determine, but the answers are there if you look. Is the evidence based on controlled scientific studies published in a peer-reviewed scientific journal, or better yet, a meta-analysis or systematic review of multiple studies? This is the best evidence available, and this is the type of evidence that supports existing interventions based on the principles of ABA, medication for addressing particular behaviors or co-occurring conditions, or allied health profession approaches. In contrast, is the evidence based on word of mouth or case study? Be wary of those treatments where the evidence is based on testimonials or for which the supporter states that it can't be proven scientifically. These are great examples of interventions that have zero evidence that they are effective. Realistically the evidence for the effectiveness of a treatment will be on a continuum where some approaches have a lot of evidence and others have less.

Is the Treatment Safe?

What are the side effects? What are the costs? Is the treatment potentially harmful? Does investing in this treatment prevent you from engaging in a treatment that is more effective, thereby having an outcome of a net loss?

Plotting Your Answers

The next step is to plot the answer to these three questions in a grid (see the diagram on the following page). The first step is to get a sense if the treatment makes sense. If so, you can move to evaluate the effectiveness and safety. The interaction among these three questions (Does it make sense? Is it effective? Is it safe?) can help guide your decision making. Of course, the recommended treatments that will fall into the top right quadrant of the figure, such as behaviorally based and allied health profession interventions, are those that have strong evidence in support of their effectiveness and safety and should form the lion's share of your treatment package. As we've already discussed, the medications used to address challenging behaviors, while effective, also have side effects. These types of medications would fall into the bottom right quadrant: strong evidence of effectiveness but information indicating the presence of side effects.

Does the intervention make sense?
- What does the treatment do?
- Is there a theory behind the approach?
- How does the treatment address your child's autism symptoms?
- Whom is it designed to help?
- Whom does it not work for?

NO, it doesn't seem to make sense.

YES, it seems to make sense.

Do not include as part of your treatment package.

How effective is the intervention?

		Limited Evidence	Strong Evidence
How safe is the intervention?	Strong Evidence	You could use cautiously and closely monitor for effectiveness.	This is recommended treatment. As always, continue to monitor for safety and effectiveness for your child.
	Limited Evidence	You should avoid this type of treatment.	You could consider, but use extreme caution and closely monitor for safety.

Is the Treatment a Good Fit for Your Family?

This question doesn't rely on any evidence or scientific input. It doesn't require any research or consultation with your physician. This question relies on your sense of whether the treatment will or won't work for your family. Not all interventions will work with every family, so finding the right fit is critical. Science shows that if a treatment isn't a good fit, the individual or family won't invest in it (e.g., won't consistently take the pill or won't attend the therapy session), and if that happens, the treatment just won't be effective.

For example, does having a professional come into your home day in and day out not fit with your family culture? Perhaps the idea of having a behavioral therapist sitting in your living room three afternoons a week with your child is not tenable for your family. If not, consider alternatives that achieve the same goals. Ideally, you could identify another setting where the intervention can occur with the same frequency and intensity and opportunities for generalizing the skills learned to your child's natural environment. Relatedly, is the treatment affordable? Some interventions can be very costly, and there are other family needs to consider. If an intervention is not affordable, there may be ways to reach those goals with a combination of different, less costly approaches. In this case, cost of the treatment may be a deciding factor.

When an intervention is a good fit for your family, you'll stay committed to it. Staying committed to treatment regimens can be tiring, but for a treatment to be effective, it has to be administered the appropriate way. If you don't think you can administer the treatment appropriately, you won't reap the benefits and won't be able to determine whether it's actually working. So, selecting components of your treatment package that you support and can maintain is an important step in seeing that treatment through.

PUTTING IT ALL TOGETHER

You've gotten an evaluation. You've identified your child's strengths and weaknesses and from that identified treatment approaches to build on those strengths and address those challenges. You've then been given the challenging job of being communication expert, services ringleader, and tirelessly persistent advocate. You've become an overnight expert on autism treatments and carefully evaluated the various treatment options that are available. Based on all this you have assembled a treatment package that relies heavily on evidence-based practices, you've prioritized the approaches, and you've promoted communication and integration of goals across providers and school, and then you begin. And then what?

Then you observe what happens. You'll want to pay attention and examine the impact of the interventions. Are skills improving? Are skills staying the same? Are there any side effects? Are there unintended consequences for the rest of the family? The answers to these questions help determine when to revise your treatment package. There will be times when skills seem to improve and then plateau and then improve again. When the improvement stagnates and the plateau extends, it is time to change the package. That might mean another evaluation with a provider to examine your child's strengths and weaknesses. It might mean a simple consultation with your physician. Or it might mean it is time to add in another recommended treatment.

There may be times when your child achieves the established goals. When that happens, it's time to establish new goals, keep using the approaches that have been working, and toss out the approaches that haven't been effective. Or, to make things more complex, previously ineffective strategies may be more appropriate now, and so you can reintroduce those previously tried approaches. The important point is to keep on evaluating and revising your treatment package.

Just as there is no one treatment that is effective for all children with autism, there is no one treatment that is effective for a child's whole life. Your job as the ringmaster will be to carefully observe when changes occur and determine when tweaks to the treatment package are needed. As your child progresses through school, different challenges may emerge, requiring different approaches. As your child transitions into adolescence, the neurodevelopmental changes that take place during those teenage years may necessitate new strategies and approaches. And as your child moves into adulthood, you may be met with new challenges that require new solutions.

By taking the new science of autism with you on your journey, you'll be able to ensure that you're on the correct path. And when you stray, as we all do, you'll be able to hop right back on that path. By applying what we know about evidence-based approaches and the new science of diet, exercise, and sleep, you will be able to help your child reach his potential.

◈

Take-Home Points

- Make sure that the provider or team that conducts your child's diagnostic evaluation informs and guides the development of your child's individualized treatment package. The recommendations need to be specific to your child's unique challenges and strengths.

- Scientific consensus is that the diagnostic evaluation should entail both caregiver interview and direct observation of your child and may include additional components as needed, such as assessment of cognitive abilities and a neurological exam.

- Your role as ringmaster of the treatment package is to coordinate its components, promote communication, be persistent in your role as advocate, and take care of yourself. Science has shown that parents of children with autism have heightened levels of stress. Heightened stress is associated with poorer outcomes. Self-care is critical to reducing stress and improving outcomes.

- The interventions with demonstrated effectiveness based on scientific study that may be part of your treatment package include therapies based on ABA; speech, occupational, or physical therapies; and medications to address related symptoms such as disruptive behavior, hyperactivity, or anxiety.

- There are hundreds of complementary and alternative treatments proposed to treat autism that have limited or no empirical evidence. A helpful framework to evaluate these treatments is to balance risk with strength of evidence. A risky treatment requires very strong evidence. A safe and healthy treatment requires a lower level of evidence to justify trying it. Later in this book, we will be discussing some of these treatments, such as those to address sleep issues, in more detail.

6

EXERCISE, SLEEP, AND ASD

Science now recognizes the brain is malleable and "plastic." That means the brain can to a surprising extent "reinvent itself" with learning, experience, or the right stimulation. We also now know that changes in gene expression (i.e., epigenetic changes) in the brain help it do that. The limits on this ability remain open frontiers for investigation, but the possibilities bring hope. As a result, we're experiencing an explosion of scientific interest in whether we can promote skills such as social behaviors, attention and executive function, even self-regulation and behavioral control, by stimulating changes in gene expression in the brain. How far can we go with changes in lifestyle that also might stimulate epigenetic change? It turns out that two major lifestyle activities that also affect general health are particularly relevant to promoting exactly the parts of the brain that strengthen self-regulation and executive function, two critical cognitive abilities that impact day-to-day functioning, and thus can help improve outcomes and increase quality of life in ASD. Those activities are exercise and sleep. Getting exercise and getting enough sleep are obviously good for general health and good for all children. But for kids with ASD, they may have specific benefits that are well worth your time to understand and consider for your own child. And sleep is particularly critical for individuals with autism. As you likely know from your personal experience and what the scientific literature tells us, most individuals with autism struggle with sleep problems at some point in their lives.

EXERCISE

The benefits of exercise and overall fitness are well established for general health, mood, and stress management. These perks are increasingly popularized in the media. For example, earlier this year the *Washington Post* published a story on exercise as "medicine"—highlighting that exercise can be an effective intervention for many health conditions. But what is the real benefit for children, in particular for those with ASD? How important is this particular lifestyle option? With the advent of studies that combine exercise and brain imaging, we're learning exactly what exercise can do for brain growth. And recent studies have just started to determine to what extent exercise can help children with ASD. While these are early days, the future is likely to bring further positive evidence.

Particularly interesting for ASD in recent years is a series of findings showing that for developing children, some forms of exercise expand the growth of brain connections, the frontal cortex, and the brain chemicals (such as serotonin and dopamine) that support self-regulation and executive functioning. These surprisingly specific findings in typically developing children have led to real excitement about the possibility that the right kind of exercise can help ASD. We'll dig into this evidence, evaluate it, and sort out what kind of exercise is best based on the findings of just the last 5 years.

What Do We Mean by "Exercise"?

First, let's talk terms: What do we mean by "exercise"? While exercise is highly beneficial, what we call "free play" has its own inherent benefits independent of any exercise. Recent findings confirm that free play helps children develop problem solving, coping skills, imagination, and self-directed learning. For preschool children, most free play involves large-motor activity and so is ideal for their development. However, for school-age children, free play is often less active, though it remains just as important for other reasons. We know that initiating, organizing, and sustaining free play, developing imaginative games, or engaging in play with other children can be difficult for many children with ASD. Yet with structure and guidance healthy forms of free play can be modeled and then taught. Gradually, the supports can then be removed so that free play can happen more independently for a child with ASD.

Sports, likewise, have a different set of benefits. They may provide exercise, although this varies with the sport. They can also provide naturalistic opportunities for practicing and improving social abilities and, for children with ASD who are good at the sport, provide an inclusive community and engagement with peers. For some children with ASD, these opportunities can help promote positive self-image to offset their struggles in social interactions in general. However, for others with ASD who are not so gifted or inclined, or who may have struggles with motor abilities or peer acceptance, sports can be an extremely frustrating and unhappy experience. As with so much else involved in helping children with ASD, it's important to know what each individual child or teen can handle and enjoy. Later in this chapter, we'll give some examples of how different types of sports experiences can provide exercise while also reinforcing the social skills that kids with ASD need to build.

Either way, sports that involve a lot of waiting may not do enough for the brain or for fitness or be a good fit for your child with autism. Some sports are great for fitness: one-on-one racquetball, basketball, soccer, high-activity dancing, bicycling, running—in these sports there's plenty of vigorous exercise and often mental challenge as well. In contrast, just playing nine-on-nine baseball, golfing with a cart, or eleven-on-eleven American football might not bring enough fitness, unless accompanied by a practice regimen that enforces fitness. Further, the social aspect of these sports may not be rewarding or may be too challenging for your child, reducing the likelihood of the sport being a successful venture.

> Exercise, sports, and free play all have particular benefits, and where fitness is concerned it's important to know what will work best for your unique child with ASD.

Keep in mind that children's fitness habits can stay with them into adulthood. If you played soccer throughout your childhood and adolescence, you might very well seek out an adult soccer league to play in. But for most adults, team sports are logistically challenging. That's why most adults in our society stay fit through individual exercise. For all children, exercise is a good habit to instill early in life, not just because cardio and strength/flexibility training will be key to adult health, but because in childhood cognitive and motor development work in tandem. In the brain, extensive connections wire motor centers, like the cerebellum and the motor cortex, to areas involved in attention and executive functioning, like the prefrontal cortex and the basal ganglia. Some physiologists believe that for the best cognitive and self-regulation outcomes for kids, exercise should include cognitive challenge, complex motor learning, and coordination in real-world conditions—that is, general motor skill growth along with aerobic challenge. Others believe the key is to combine physical effort with cognitive challenge, as on the soccer field or basketball court. For preschoolers, this may occur naturally through running, climbing, organizing games, or wrestling around during free play. But for older children, it may require an organized activity, either individually or with a partner or a team. These might include activities like rock climbing, dance, basketball, or martial arts. Here again, you'll have to use some judgment to balance free play and structured activity, mental and emotional engagement and fitness challenge. If your teenager is rock climbing (with a qualified supervisor) during free play, her free play and ideal exercise may be one and the same. On the other hand, if your 10-year-old is using his free play time to build a model with Legos or to read, then he may need, in addition, to go for a vigorous bike ride or play a sport.

In addition, if your child with ASD has experience in a sporting activity, it provides a structured opportunity to practice and develop social skills. This continues to be critical throughout an individual's life. Early in life, a group-based exercise activity will provide a fertile ground to develop new interactive and reciprocal social skills. Later in life, exercise provides an opportunity to remain engaged in the community. This becomes increasingly essential for adults with autism, who may finish with school and need community activities that are rewarding and successful. Think of promoting exercise and sport-based skills as similar to giving your child a talent like playing the piano or your young adult a job. Having a skill as a child or a job as an adult promotes opportunities for social interactions, which for autism are absolutely critical to ongoing development. In turn, all those social opportunities, provided they are successful and scaffolded appropriately, can lay the groundwork for stronger neural networks underlying social abilities.

Choosing the Best Exercise

Before we focus on ASD-related exercise benefits, it's important to put them in the context of these guidelines:

1. Group sports should be considered optional, and decisions made about enrolling your child in a specific sports program should be based on the following, in this order:

- *Your child's ability to meet the social, communicative, and organizational demands of the sport with the supports that are available.* This may limit the options for your child, but advocating for the specific supports that your child needs may open up more opportunities.

- *Your child's ability to enjoy the sport.* If your child is thriving in a particular sport, encourage it. If she hates it, let her do something else. Many children with autism enjoy the structure of some martial arts. Others enjoy individual sports, like running. For some children, sports have very limited interest. Special interests that your child has may interfere with the development of interest in sports, but using those interests as a reward for participation may increase the likelihood your child will try out new activities.

- *The level of vigorous exercise (breathing harder, heart rate up)*

2. Always allow your child with ASD enough time for healthy forms of free play (active or not), adding exercise on top of free play if necessary. Given the often full days of intervention that many children with autism have, adding exercise may be too much and may not be appropriate.

3. The main thing is to get the exercise, which can be done in a lot of different ways. Stay open.

Exercise, Epigenetics, and the Brain

Exercise is a lifestyle factor with some of the clearest epigenetic effects. A sustained fitness program, at any age, causes significant epigenetic changes throughout the body, both in obvious locations like heart and muscle genes, and, it turns out, also in the brain. The brain growth effects, under study for the past several years, now have a sufficiently large literature to be considered definite. They were confirmed in comprehensive scientific reviews in 2013 and 2014 and additional reviews in 2016 and 2017.

The epigenetic effects on the brain are still being studied, but evidence so far is quite positive. Animal studies suggest that exercise triggers epigenetic changes that specifically alter activity in genes that influence new neuron growth and extend neural dendritic connections. In plain English, this means that exercise can exert effects that make the brain grow and become more efficient. Even more encouraging regarding ASD is that this seems to happen in particular brain areas like the hippocampus, basal ganglia, and frontal cortex that, as discussed in previous chapters, have been implicated in ASD and are fundamental to learning, self-regulation, and executive functioning. In these animal studies mice either exercise vigorously or do not, and then are examined for brain growth, gene expression, and epigenetic changes. Do such animal studies prove that children who exercise will get the same benefits? It's a bit of a stretch, but actually it doesn't get much better than this as far as effects we would want to see in an animal model go. So these studies, while preliminary, are quite encouraging. Let's look at the effects of exercise on children in three areas relevant to ASD: learning, attention, and ASD symptoms, specifically.

Exercise and Learning/Attention

Kids with ASD can face a variety of obstacles to academic learning, ranging from difficulties with transitions to problems managing social interactions to struggles with intellectual delays. For some children with autism these challenges will drive academic problems. However, as we mentioned briefly in Chapter 1, most children with autism also have problems with attention and executive function and difficulties associated with ADHD, and these are some of the biggest obstacles to academic learning. Therefore, an important area for us to look at with exercise is whether it helps kids with their academics, and in particular with the executive function part of academic success.

Fortunately, developmental studies of child exercise have used academic results as a primary focus (in part because school physical education programs make it a natural place to do safe, controlled experiments). Despite this, the caveat is that this literature is still short on very-high-quality randomized trials of the sort that provide the acid test of exercise benefits. Thus, we have to make inferences from studies with various limits. However, in just the past year countless reviews of the data in other studies of typically developing children highlight the important finding that exercise has significant and positive benefits on learning, memory, and executive functioning skills. A major monograph published in 2014 by the Society for Research in Child Development concluded that overall, real-world exercise led to improved academic performance in children—more than equivalent additional class or study time. In other words, school policies to cut physical education classes are a mistake. The science indicates that schools should convert physical education classes into physical fitness classes and keep them going. We definitely need more randomized trials to gain confidence here, but if we try to peer into the future, the most likely picture is that exercise improves learning, attention, and executive functioning in typically developing children, and therefore it's reasonable to suppose that it directly assists with challenges often associated with ASD by building self-regulation in the brain.

Until the 2010s, we had no direct data, however, on whether ASD itself would improve with exercise. Now such data is finally emerging, albeit slowly.

Exercise and Core Symptoms of ASD: Social Skills and Repetitive Behaviors

More than a dozen studies to date have focused on evaluating whether children with ASD benefit from an exercise program. Unfortunately, these studies are all very small and riddled with inconsistency and methodological limitations, so this is not yet a "mature" literature that allows confident conclusions. Still, we can see some trends that are important. A 2016 statistical summary of all studies found 22 small studies evaluating the impact of exercise on cognition in 579 people between 3 and 35 years of age with ASD or ADHD. Importantly, only six of those studies were conducted with children with ASD, totaling 128 children, and while the investigators' determined diagnosis did not impact the effect of the intervention on outcomes, the majority of the information from this summary comes from studies of children with ADHD, not ASD. However, with that caution in mind, the pooled data were still encouraging: overall there is a small but significant positive benefit of physical exercise on aspects of cognition. That is, exercise-based interventions have a positive impact on cognitive abilities—specifically the ability to maintain attention or to stay on task. Given the problems with self-regulation that are part of autism, this finding provides hope.

Between 2016 and 2017, two systematic reviews attempted to quantify the evidence for the benefits of exercise programs as a treatment for the core challenges of ASD, including social deficits, repetitive behaviors, self-regulation, and cognition. These reviews focused on children with ASD younger than 16 years for one study and younger than 21 years for the second. The reviews revealed that the vast majority of the individual studies reviewed were flawed in some way. For example, the hypotheses were not always clearly stated, and inclusion criteria were unclear, but both reviews did conclude that there was moderate evidence for the effectiveness of physical exercise on improving behavioral outcomes (specifically, reduction of repetitive behaviors), social–emotional functioning, attention, and cognition.

Caveats: What We Still Don't Know

- *Which kinds of exercises don't help the brain?* Most research has been on cardio (aerobic) exercise and often in a laboratory that doesn't involve a real-world goal (thus omitting the learning, motivation, and engagement that may be part of the holistic benefits of exercise). What about strength training or other types of exercise? Work on this is just beginning.

- *How permanent are benefits in children?* Most studies are on adults, often on older adults, and most experimental trials with children have been pretty limited.

- *While the research demonstrating exercise benefits on cognition is strong, how consistent is the impact on social skills development?* The limited and often flawed available research suggests there is potential benefit, but we need more research in this area.

- *What is the sustained benefit of fitness programs (as opposed to same-day or same-week benefit) for kids with ASD?* This has not yet been studied.

- *How big are individual differences?* Should different kids with different genetic makeups have different kinds of exercise to maximize their brain growth and attention? This new area is important to study. Like everything else in this book, the answer won't end up being one size fits all. A particular question is whether boys and girls benefit from the same activities; most studies to date have been on boys.

• *How long should you continue the fitness program to help support your child with ASD?* We don't know, but we can infer some principles from the literature. One is that even as little as a week can help—but then only temporarily. Longer effort is likely to yield longer-term benefits. And even though exercise causes epigenetic changes, it takes sustained exercise over time for those to build up to a noticeable influence on growth. Growing the brain is like growing the muscles—it requires sustained fitness, suggesting you should maintain the effort over several weeks or months.

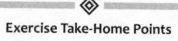

Exercise Take-Home Points

- If your child has ASD, the benefits of exercise are even more important than for other kids. The unique effects of exercise on the brain networks and gene expression patterns that support maturation of self-regulation should make you sit up and take notice.

- Exercise and fitness have a nice side effect of protecting your child from serious health problems (like obesity and diabetes), improving health in such areas as skin, muscle, and bone, and improving coordination. Initial studies also show that exercise may have positive effects on your child's social skills, reduce repetitive behaviors, and improve self-regulation and cognition by supporting brain growth in systems that underlie these abilities. This will improve quality of life for your child with ASD.

- With epigenetic effects involved, developmental effects may well be sustained even during years that exercise slacks off—we are still learning how many effects are short term versus long term in this regard.

- A final benefit shown in studies is that exercise is a powerful route to creating epigenetic change that can overcome negative events earlier in life. For example, animal studies have reported that exercise can prevent or reverse the epigenetic effects of stress and trauma in early life.

- Exercise can be fun—it's sometimes a matter of finding the right outlet to pique your child's interest. For some families, it helps to exercise with your child—a shared bike ride, hike, run, or game.

- Exercise may be most beneficial when combined with any special interests your child may have. By building on his unique interests or preoccupations you can foster a healthier physical lifestyle while capitalizing on what is most reinforcing for him. For example, there was a young man I (Bernier) used to work with whose love of monitoring steps on his Fitbit led him to the hobby of long-distance running. He would tally his steps at the end of each day and chart out his progress. The running part was an afterthought to him, but provided him with excellent health benefits.

Exercise Action Steps

On several occasions in the past decade, scientists have surveyed the landscape for typically developing children. Lacking ASD-specific guidelines, our best bet is to go with these general guidelines but to highlight their likely extra relevance to children with ASD, who need every boost they can get in relation to social development, learning, executive function, and self-regulation. That being said, we recognize that some of these recommendations may be very challenging to achieve for your child. Please do not be discouraged. If they don't work at this time for your family, keep them in mind for the future. Here are the general and most common recommendations.

- *Help your child get at least 1 hour a day of moderate and moderate-to-intensive exercise (heart rate up and breathing a bit harder).* It doesn't have to be all at once. It can be one 60-minute period, two 30-minute periods, or four 15-minute periods. (These guidelines come from the American Heart Association.) Some children need more exercise than others. Some children may be happier and calmer if they can get 2 hours a day, but even some exercise will help their health and mood. Some children (whether they have autism or not) may be unwilling to exercise. Reward charts, token systems, or other reinforcement programs can be put in place, as with any other behavior you'd like to encourage. Sticker charts displayed on the refrigerator may be an appropriate reinforcer to encourage young children to complete some physical activity, while working toward a goal over a period of a week or two (such as an activity with Dad or a small prize) may be appropriate for a teenager with sufficient cognitive and self-regulatory skills.

• *If realistically feasible, try for the main exercise at the beginning of the day so your child is ready for the school day.* While this is difficult to arrange, some schools and some families have been able to do it. It's the ideal! However, obviously that won't be possible for everyone. Most kids will have to go to school and then get their exercise after school, in addition to what we all hope is recess time. Weekend mornings are often a good time for families to get out and walk in a park or play at a playground. Doing that in the beginning of the day often promotes more physical activity.

• *Aim for the exercise to include a mix of moderate activity (walking, level bicycling, roller blading, skateboarding, jumping rope, playing on the playground) and moderate to intense activity* sufficient to make the child huff and puff or break a sweat (running, cycling on hills, swimming, vigorous dancing, martial arts, soccer, basketball, playing chase, gymnastics, sustained calisthenics). (These recommendations come from the British National Health Service.) The activity should be consistent during the time period—don't count activities that include a lot of standing around or waiting for a turn.

• *Include activities that involve motor skill learning and coordination*—that is, some cognitive challenge. While the extra benefits of this approach are not yet definitive, it is possible that added brain growth happens here. Most ball sports involve at least some motor learning, while dance, martial arts, rock climbing, gymnastics, cross-fit, or some calisthenics like jump rope may entail more complete whole-body muscle learning. It's precisely because many forms of exercise require motor skills and coordination that children with autism, who are more likely to have minor motor delays or challenges, often will not be drawn to exercise and sports. But you can treat sports and exercise as behavioral therapies to support social skills development in which social skills are trained and reinforced. By following your child's lead on any interests in physical activity and reinforcing participation in those activities with rewards, you can over time promote more interest and skill in physical fitness.

• *It's OK to mix activities.* You don't have to hit all aspects every day. For example, your child may like to run sometimes and play soccer or basketball other times, or to dance a couple times a week and go bike riding other times. However, your child with autism may have more narrow interests, and it's OK to follow her lead if she's interested in one particular form of exercise. The aim here is to support physical fitness in whatever way is appropriate for your family.

• *Include free play if exercise is all structured.* School-age kids should get an hour of free play and an hour of good exercise—that's two hours if the free play is not moderate to vigorous exercise. For your child, as with many children with autism, free play may not be a successful activity. If structured exercise is the only way to engage your child physically, by all means, focus on that.

• *Finally, don't be too hard on yourself if you can't hit the ideals—* some exercise for your child is better than none. A few ideas from parents who have been there can be found below.

Ideas for Meeting the Exercise Challenge

For many families, fitting in exercise is a real challenge, depending on their child's needs and abilities, the climate, cost, and neighborhood. It may prove necessary to have different activities in summer and winter. While organized school or community sports after school work for many families, they aren't for all. Here are some examples of other solutions families have found:

• Kim went for runs while her son rode his bike on weekend days because he loved riding his bike.

• Michael enrolled in Aikido with his daughter so that he could support her success in a group activity and promote her social interactions.

• Bill supported additional time for his son's para-educator to join him on the field during his team's soccer games so Bill Jr. could practice social skills and move his body on the field.

• Nome organized obstacle courses on the playground for her daughter with ASD and her typically developing son and timed them with a stopwatch. The timing structure helped her daughter stay engaged in the activity and get excited about matching their own "world record" time.

• Jennifer enrolled her daughter in the nonprofit Girls on the Run and found the exercise helped combat the weight-gain side effects of her medication (see Chapter 5 for more on medication).

SLEEP

Knowledge regarding the relationship between sleep, another major lifestyle consideration, and ASD has expanded rapidly. It turns out that many children with autism have sleep problems of one sort or another. In fact, more kids with autism have problems falling asleep than not. This may not surprise you: for years parents reported challenges with sleep for their children with autism, yet the scientific and provider community was slow to respond. Fortunately, the last 10 years have seen considerable focus on sleep problems in autism and the development of tools to address those challenges. Part of the drive for this focus in autism is the recent gains in our understanding of sleep's importance broadly and the availability of many tools that can be adapted to improve sleep for children with autism. Importantly, improving sleep can actually boost your child's self-regulation and brain development. The science has a lot to tell us about sleep and brain development, and in this section we'll explain how significant these findings are for your child with ASD.

Chances are you don't get enough sleep and neither do your kids. National surveys indicate that 70% of teens and 70% of adults are not getting enough sleep.

Sleep problems are very common in children, whether the child has autism or not. In one recent national survey, over half of parents reported their child had some sort of sleep problem, and one-fourth of parents reported their child did not get enough sleep. As we'll describe below, the rates of sleep problems for children with autism are even higher. Based on the prevalence of sleep issues, some of the co-occurrence of ASD and sleep problems is just the random overlap of two common problems. However, let's dig deeper as there is more than just randomness. There are causal connections.

During sleep, the brain grows new connections, stores memories, and repairs cells. One striking scientific finding is called sleep-dependent memory consolidation, or sleep-dependent learning. This means it's during sleep that learning takes hold. You may be all too familiar with the common complaint in ASD that a child seems to learn something one day but then has to learn it all over again the next day. This is an example of failure of memory consolidation. The fact is that children can't learn things if they don't sleep! And many things that may come easily to a typically developing child, such as how to make sense of facial expressions or how to have a conversation, will require additional cognitive effort for your child with autism. Meaning that if your child is not sleeping, it is even more difficult for her to learn those needed social skills.

Sleep is also crucial to managing stress and emotions and to having the mental capacity for focused attention. The ability of your child to manage the stress of navigating social situations, filter out sensory stimuli, and attend in class (often all at the same time), will be significantly impacted by the quantity and quality of his sleep.

Sleep seems to be nature's number-one tool for growing a child's brain.

As the brain is developing, it uses sleep in different distinct ways in early life. Infants use sleep to generalize from one experience to another. Their naps play a crucial role in learning. Recent experiments have shown that babies exposed to new learning remember it if they have napped in between the tests, but not if they stayed awake. Preschoolers use sleep to retain specific things they learned during the day. Children, teens, and adults continue to use sleep to lock in learning. In recent years, studies like those just mentioned have clarified, in animals and humans, that children and adults learn just as much asleep as while awake. As with babies, when they see new information, they remember it better if they sleep before the memory test than if they don't. Brain-imaging studies using magnetic resonance imaging (MRI) detect patterns of brain activation that show something remarkable: a particular brain pattern activates when seeing new information awake, and the same pattern is replayed during sleep. This indicates that during sleep the brain works to consolidate and store what it learned in the daytime.

Now sleep scientists do not see sleep as merely helpful in child learning—they see it as necessary. In fact, some recent studies suggest that children who sleep more have higher IQs, as well as better attention and self-control—all very relevant if your child has ASD! Max is a 10-year-old minimally verbal boy with autism who regularly came in to my (Bernier's) clinic to work on his aggressive outbursts following frustrating events, such as when transitioning from preferred activities to tasks at school or after unexpected changes to his routine. After several weeks of behavioral treatment, Max's rate of aggressive outbursts settled to a consistent rate of about twice per week, down from twice a day. A few weeks later Max's father came back to the clinic because the rate of aggressive outbursts had risen to twice a day again. Although there had been no unexpected changes to his routine or schedule, some careful investigation revealed that Max was not sleeping well after having been an excellent sleeper. He was still following his sleep routines to a T, but now he was lying in bed for nearly an hour before falling asleep. Through some remarkable detective work, Max's parents found out that this was happening because one of Max's shades had broken and light from a streetlight was coming in. Max's father replaced the shade, Max returned to falling asleep almost immediately, and the rate of his aggressive outbursts dropped back down. Sleep was significantly impacting Max's self-control.

Sleep, Genetics, and Epigenetics

Our circadian rhythms, the rhythms generated by our brain that approximate the length of a day and night, are regulated by many factors, with genetics playing a role. Animal models have shown us that there are several genes associated with circadian rhythms and sleep. These "clock genes" help maintain our circadian rhythms and impact our sleep–wake cycles. Some studies suggest that in ASD rare versions of these clock genes are observed more often, the clock genes may function differently, and that there are higher rates of mutations to these genes. However, this area of research is just emerging, so the true relationship between sleep and ASD at the genetic level is still yet to be determined.

By now you should not be surprised to find out that sleep regulation, like so many other functions, depends not just on genetics but on epigenetic signaling. For example, a study in 2015 looked at pairs of identical twins in which one twin wanted to go to sleep early in the evening and the other wanted to go to sleep later. The study found the twins had differences in epigenetic marks on certain circadian genes— implying changes in how those genes were functioning in the brain.

Evidence for ASD is limited, but one kind of circumstantial evidence is interesting. One of the genes involved in Rett syndrome (related to ASD) is also involved in circadian rhythms. The gene is called *MeCP2*. When experimenters disrupted the sleep–wake cycles in mice, they found that *MeCP2* activity had changed. This suggests that epigenetics can impact functioning of key genes associated with neurodevelopmental disorders like ASD.

Some sleep problems likely develop from early experiences that disrupt the settings of the brain's circadian clock via epigenetic change. We already know from a great deal of research that the day–night cycle sets off light-sensitive reactions in key areas of babies' brains that are part of their normal development, so babies adapt to the light–dark cycle where they live. Epigenetic changes do that coding in their young brain. If epigenetic changes early in a child's life can affect how the child sleeps, can we provide training or other experiences that will reverse a current sleep problem? We don't know for sure, but everything we've learned so far about epigenetics suggests that it's at least possible. Let's look at the best ideas for how to resolve a sleep problem.

Sleep and Autism

We don't need research studies to tell us that we can't focus, pay attention, or concentrate well without good sleep. But science adds an important detail: this problem with attention can carry over even after sleep is restored. You also know from experience that your self-control quickly stumbles after a sleepless night. You can't cope nearly as well with stress, handle your emotions, or focus when overtired. The same goes for kids, of course. In short, if your child isn't getting enough sleep, her attention and behavior may look disrupted and dysregulated. And what if your child has ASD? Here are the facts to keep in mind regarding sleep and ASD:

- Sleep is active, not passive. It's an essential part of wiring the brain and learning. Kids with ASD usually have either delays or losses in brain development, as well as problems learning, so it is fundamental for them to try to recover in these areas.

- Lack of sleep can exacerbate existing symptoms that children with

ASD show. To get a good understanding of the degree of a child's challenges, we need to make sure sleep is adequate.

- The prevalence rate of obstructive sleep apnea appears to be similar in ASD to that in the general population. The rate of restless legs syndrome appears to be somewhat higher in ASD (although it's difficult to assess). Thus, both of these disorders are less common than other causes of sleep challenges. However, they should be evaluated when management of sleep-related behaviors proves ineffective and your child still shows signs of not being rested.

- Children with ASD often have sleep-related behavior problems that interfere with getting adequate sleep.

If your child isn't getting enough sleep, or enough good-quality sleep, then you can expect inattention, disorganization, moodiness, tantrums, irritability, and health problems, from more colds to vague complaints. What's worse, your child's brain growth will not be happening under its preferred conditions. If you are like most parents, chances are decent that your kids may not be getting adequate sleep, simply by the law of averages—a substantial percentage of children (and adults) do not get adequate sleep in the United States! Our lives are often just too overloaded. Once again, many children may be able to tolerate this state of affairs without obvious ill effects. But if your child has ASD, you have less margin for error to "let this one go." Sleep is an area where it might make a lot of sense to take some action.

How Much Sleep Should Your Child Be Getting?

How much sleep developing children need may surprise you. The National Sleep Foundation recommends that from zero to 2 years of age infants and toddlers get more than 12 hours of sleep a day. Many, of course, get some of this by napping. Preschoolers need 10–13 hours (for a median of 11 hours). School-age children typically should be getting 10 hours of sleep a night (some guidelines suggest 11 hours). While there can certainly be individuals who go outside of these ranges, for most of you that means if your child has to get up at 7:00 A.M. for school, she should be asleep by 9:00 P.M., starting to get ready for bed by 8:30, and turning

Children and teens with autism need the same amounts of sleep as their typical peers, but because ASD can make sleep challenging, and the benefits of adequate sleep are even more important, a good night's sleep every night should be a priority.

off screens and ending stimulating activities by 8:00. Teens need only a little less—9 to 10 hours, depending on which guidelines one follows. With school starting at 8:00 or 8:30, early bedtimes are required.

This is very difficult for teenagers, whose biological clocks are set for a later cycle than adults by evolution. That change in their body clocks is not an aberration but a normal developmental phase of adolescence. The table below gives some sample sleep schedules based on National Sleep Foundation guidelines (*http://sleepfoundation.org*).

Sleep and Teenagers

Getting enough sleep during the teen years is a special challenge. Teens still need at least 9 hours of sleep, and 10 might be better. Yet only 30% of teens even get 8 hours of sleep per night. The challenge is particularly serious because teens naturally have later circadian clocks—they don't want to go to bed as early as adults do. Evolution has designed us that way. Ideally, teens could stay up late and sleep late—as many do in the summer and on weekends. This is natural for their development. This creates an especially difficult situation if your teen has ASD, however, because children with ASD can ill afford to lose sleep. The importance of sleep for learning and self-regulation means that your child (who will

Sample Schedules

	Target range	Median	Bedtime	Asleep	Wake
Preschool (3–5)	10–13	11.5	7:00 P.M.	7:30 P.M.	7:00 A.M.
School age (6–13)	9–11	10	8:30 P.M.	9:00 P.M.	7:00 A.M.
Teen (14–17)	8–10	9	9:30 P.M.	10:00 P.M.	7:00 A.M.
Young adult (18+)	7–9	8	10:30 P.M.	11:00 P.M.	7:00 A.M.

require extra effort to learn from the social world—even things that may be effortless for typically developing teens) will be at an even greater disadvantage if managing the social world without enough sleep.

In 2014 the American Academy of Pediatrics issued a policy statement recommending that middle and high school should not start before 8:30 A.M. Yet fewer than 20% of schools comply with this recommendation at present; the average start time nationwide is 8:00 A.M., and some start earlier. In 2015 the calls for change grew louder. An expert summary of the problem and recommendations were provided in November 2015 in *Perspectives in Psychological Science,* which recommends pushing back high school start times as late as possible. Some municipalities are actively moving in that direction, and some states have moved most of their schools to an 8:30 or later start.

In the meantime, it's normal for teens, unfortunately, to struggle to go to sleep at night and get up in the morning. For some teens this pattern does cross the line to a delayed sleep–wake phase disorder—but you need a doctor to determine if it has. According to the American Academy of Sleep Medicine, the hallmarks of a delayed sleep–wake phase disorder are (1) difficulty getting to sleep and waking up and (2) sleepiness during the day.

What's Causing the Problem?

If you know your child isn't getting enough sleep and is showing the negative effects of undersleeping, you obviously need to figure out why this is happening. For kids with ASD, sleep problems fall into two classes:

1. *Secondary sleep problems,* such as problems with bedtime. Here the problem is usually that ASD is contributing to sleep problems! Other medical conditions that we see more often in ASD can also result in insomnia and serve as secondary sleep problems. We often see gastrointestinal problems in ASD, and both constipation and reflux can make lying down and staying asleep uncomfortable. Children with ASD have higher rates of seizures. Some seizures can occur more often during sleep or can be exacerbated by lack of sleep, which will impact the child's ability to fall or stay asleep. Additionally, anxiety, which is diagnosed in up to 40% of individuals with ASD, can lead to hyperarousal. Hyperarousal certainly impacts sleep, and some antianxiety medications have been shown to have a paradoxical effect for some children with ASD and increase insomnia.

2. *Primary sleep problems,* such as biological sleep–wake cycle problems or obstructive sleep apnea. Here the sleep problems may be exacerbating your child's ASD symptoms, such as difficulties managing changes to routines, repetitive behaviors, and social reciprocity, as well as associated behaviors such as poor concentration, low energy, and irritability. Of course, some children have both types of problems.

Researchers have three basic methods for studying sleep in children, listed in the box below. You can pursue one of these with a professional, but if you think your child has a sleep problem, our recommendation is to start simple and just look at bedtime routines and sleep hygiene and attack the problem behaviorally. If the following remedies for secondary sleep problems don't help, that's the time to go further with clinical evaluation and treatment.

How Sleep Problems Are Assessed by a Professional

- A short questionnaire (one is called the Children's Sleep Habits Questionnaire) or a sleep diary.

- A small motion sensor the size of a watch that is worn on the wrist or ankle. It tracks nighttime or 24-hour activity and provides a rough gauge as to when a child is asleep.

- Polysomnography—that is, an overnight sleep study in a lab where the child is attached to electrodes that monitor sleep quality (brain waves) and breathing and other measures directly. This is the "gold standard" but expensive, and only sometimes warranted.

- Additional methods of sleep tracking using sensors and smartphones are emerging but not yet very dependable for clinical purposes. Use these with caution with children due to concerns about effects of blue screens on sleep, which we'll talk about shortly.

Secondary Sleep Problems: Bedtime and Sleep Hygiene

Knowing your child's ideal sleep schedule is the easy part. Creating a calm, successful bedtime routine is a lot more challenging for most parents. If you have a child with ASD, he may be particularly resistant to bedtime because of a difficulty with transitions or with self-regulation and settling down. And because he's tired, he may escalate and have a tantrum right when you are trying to bring the day to a quiet end—and you're tired too! You have stuff to do. It can be very frustrating.

Here are the most common behavioral sleep problems recognized by the American Academy of Sleep Medicine. Although these problems are not indicators of ASD, they are more common in children with the condition. So especially if your child has ASD, you may recognize some of these.

- Falling asleep is an extended process that requires special conditions. And without the special conditions in place, the child takes a long time to go to sleep or has other sleep disruptions. Research has shown consistently that over half of all children with ASD resist bedtime and have a hard time falling asleep.

- Sleep-onset associations are highly problematic or demanding— that is, the child doesn't like to go to sleep.

- Parasomnias, like sleepwalking and nightmares, occur in approximately 50% of children with ASD.

- Nighttime awakenings require caregiver intervention for the child to return to sleep and morning arising problems create challenges for starting the day.

- Limit-setting problems occur:
  - The child has difficulty initiating or maintaining sleep.
  - The child stalls or refuses to go to bed at an appropriate time.
  - The child refuses to return to bed following a nighttime awakening.

The first line of defense to either prevent or overcome these types of problems is to establish basic "sleep hygiene"—the behavioral routine that makes sleep easier, including the bedtime routine. Let's go over that first.

The core of a good sleep hygiene routine is to have time before bed to prepare the body for sleep. This means that for at least an hour before bedtime your child should avoid blue light (computer, TV, and device screens—see the action steps on page 167), large meals, and exercise. That's the time boundary. There is also a space boundary: Keep the bed only for sleeping. (For adults it is advised to keep the whole bedroom only for sleep, but for most families this isn't possible for chil-

> Blue screens are a threat to sleep quality and should be avoided for at least an hour before bed. This includes mobile phones.

dren, whose bedrooms often double as playrooms and study rooms. But try to keep the bed for sleep only.) And as you probably know, it can be problematic and disruptive to sleep hygiene to keep a TV in the bedroom.

Is the Cell Phone or iPad Causing Your Child's Sleep Problems?

Kids with ASD love their electronics—video games, cell phones, computers, tablets, and TV. One speculation about why kids in general like these things so much is that the frequent changes in stimulation probably help keep dopamine active in the brain. Dopamine is a neurotransmitter in the brain that is involved in the reward system. The same could be said for children with ASD. Unfortunately, these devices can interfere with social development, as it's difficult to engage with others with one's face glued to a screen. Here there's another concern—the "blue light" they emit interferes with sleep.

Several studies in the past few years have confirmed what many clinicians long suspected. Children and adults who use mobile phones, computers, or televisions before going to bed sleep more poorly. When daylight dims the body naturally begins to produce melatonin to prepare for sleep. We now know that the blue light of backlit electronic screens is just the right wavelength to suppress that melatonin production. Studies using hourly saliva samples in children and adults confirm dramatic suppression of melatonin when light from the screens is reaching the eyes. Other studies using randomized controlled designs confirm that electronic screen use in the hour before bed causes insomnia (meaning it's harder to fall asleep), changes in sleep stages (such as REM sleep), and less alertness the next day.

For example, in 2015 researchers in Boston reported striking findings about using e-readers or iPads (or similar devices) compared to reading a print book during the last hour before bed. Those who used the electronic reader were less sleepy, took longer to fall asleep, had later circadian timing (including changes in melatonin and changes in REM sleep), and were less alert the next morning. Those were young adults. The same is now observed in children using a simple correlational design. In 2015, a different group (also in Boston) surveyed over 2,000 fourth- and seventh-graders. Children who slept near a small screen (including sleeping near their phone), played computer games in the evening, or had TV in their room had less sleep and felt less rested.

Behavioral Approaches to Fixing Sleep Problems

The behavioral sleep problems listed above can occur in any child but seem to be practically epidemic in children with ASD. There are as many possible reasons for this as there are children with ASD. One reason may be related to hyperarousal and the resultant difficulty in settling down to sleep. Children with autism have an increased state of arousal compared to their peers. This state of high arousal has a number of effects that can make it hard to fall asleep—from sensory sensitivities to anxiety and a decrease in melatonin, which is involved in the sleep/wake cycle—and end in frustration and negative associations with bedtime. One key concept, then, is to replace the negative experiences over time with very positive ones—making bedtime a really rewarding experience for the child. For many children with autism, this rewarding experience may simply be a specific routine. Given that difficulties with transitions are part and parcel of autism, routines are the perfect antidote to stress (and arousal) at bedtime.

Because transitions can be so difficult for children with autism, a consistent bedtime routine can prevent stress and make it easier to fall asleep.

A recent analysis of eight different reviews, which captured 38 intervention trials to tackle sleep problems in ASD, indicates that no single approach is effective across all the sleep problems observed in children with ASD. The conclusion of this systematic review, however, is that behavioral interventions, parent education program interventions, and melatonin appear to be the most effective at improving multiple types of sleep problems compared with other interventions (see the box on page 166 for more on melatonin). What makes this complicated in ASD are the varying types of sleep problems (difficulty falling asleep, difficulty staying asleep, night wake-ups, etc.).

Most professionals believe that sleep problems should first be addressed by improving sleep hygiene. If problems persist, then the use of melatonin should be considered. In trials for individuals with ASD, melatonin showed the strongest effectiveness for decreasing the time to fall asleep, increasing sleep duration, and decreasing bedtime resistance. Behavioral interventions appear to be most effective for reducing early-morning waking and co-sleeping. Parent education programs are most effective at reducing night awakening and increasing self-settling. In all cases, a physician should consider whether any medical issues, such as sleep apnea, GI problems, or seizures, could be contributing to sleep problems.

The reason for the effectiveness of parent education and behavioral interventions is probably obvious to you—implementing a new sleep schedule is not easy, and you may need a consistent, carefully designed behavior management program to make it work. See the action steps on the next page for the basics, but note that you may need to get a pro to guide you through setting up the behavioral programs and troubleshooting. The good news: the counseling need not be very intensive. A recent study found improvement in sleep after parents received just two sessions of expert guidance on getting a behavioral sleep program in place.

When You Need Help with Behavioral Sleep Difficulties

Behavioral sleep difficulties often don't clear up on their own. When they go on for a long time, there is a significant danger that they'll become entrenched. Professional counselors can help you choose from among a number of possible formal behavioral training programs. These include:

- Establishing positive routines around bedtime
- Using a behavioral technique called extinction (unmodified, graduated, or with parental presence) to reduce bedtime demands

You can work with a psychologist or counselor trained in behavioral medicine to set up a simple intervention program. You can start by trying to set up a program of your own, following the action steps on page 167, if that doesn't improve matters, get professional guidance.

Should You Try Melatonin for Your Child with ASD?

• *What is melatonin?* Melatonin is a hormone that regulates the daily circadian (sleep–wake) cycle. The body makes more melatonin when it gets dark to prepare us to sleep and less when it gets light to prepare us to be awake. Melatonin is widely used to help adults with insomnia. It is a hormone, so even though it is sold over the counter, side-effect risks are real.

• *Guidance.* Use melatonin with your child only under medical supervision and after a behavioral program fails. Based on the proceedings of a consensus conference of experts in 2014, melatonin, properly dosed, can be safe and effective to help children fall asleep (shorter "sleep latency") and sleep longer. Genetic variation in how they metabolize melatonin leads to better effects at lower doses for some people. Note that many over-the-counter tablets are poor quality and may provide far too high a dose for children.

• *Does it help ASD?* It has been hypothesized that abnormal levels of melatonin play a role in the observed sleep problems in ASD. The existing literature is limited by small sample sizes and inconclusive evidence. Regardless, however, many intervention trials with melatonin have been conducted. The results show that melatonin appears to be effective in reducing the time it takes to fall asleep, but its efficacy in reducing nighttime awakenings and addressing other aspects of sleep disturbances is more variable.

• *Risks.* We don't know enough yet about whether long-term treatment with melatonin supplements is harmful to children's still-developing endocrine system. Concerns about affecting your child's development are particularly notable with infants (their bodies are still learning how to adjust sleep and melatonin to local light cycles) and teens (whose bodies are working with rapidly changing hormone levels already).

• *Side effects.* Though not usual, side effects can include waking up in the middle of the night, a morning "hangover" (feeling drowsy, headache, feeling "down"), daytime laziness, excessive sweating at night or in the day, and bedwetting.

• *The bottom line.* Melatonin can be a useful way to help restore your child to a normal sleep cycle, especially if he is diagnosed with sleep–wake phase disorder and behavior adjustments have not worked. But poor sleep hygiene, depression, or health problems can mimic a sleep–wake phase disorder, so fix sleep hygiene and get a health checkup with your pediatrician first. Because melatonin is a hormone and its interactions with normal hormone changes in developing children are not well understood, work with your doctor.

Action Steps for Good Sleep Hygiene

Basics

- No TV in the bedroom.

- Turn off and remove blue light (all screens including cell phones) for at least an hour before bedtime; no use of cell phones in the bed.

- Avoid large meals right before bedtime.

- Keep the bedroom, or at least the bed, only for sleeping; study elsewhere.

- No vigorous exercise for at least an hour before bed; keep things calm and low key.

- Set up a routine that takes 30–45 minutes.

- Keep the child moving forward during the routine; redirect as necessary.

- Conclude with a very positive ritual enjoyable to the child (for example, a story, song, or simple phrase you say together).

- End the routine with "good night" and the child in bed alone, drowsy but awake (so he doesn't think he needs you present to fall asleep the rest of the way).

Tips

- If your child calls you back or leaves the room, minimize engagement and redirect him to sleep.

- Maintain total consistency, with the same routine and schedule every night.

- The best rewards are praise and affection—keep it positive.

- Use a point or token system if you have to in order to keep the child motivated to follow the routine. This system may be more appropriate for a teenager or may be most effective if your child is motivated by tangible rewards.

- Write out the schedule if that helps the child target what you want.

- Counselors can help you create a stronger, more formal behavioral plan if needed.

Primary Sleep Disorders and ASD

In addition to getting on a good sleep schedule and practicing good sleep hygiene to address the behavioral side of sleep, sleep itself has to be good quality. Poor sleep habits like watching TV before bed can cause insomnia as well as poor quality of sleep when sleeping. However, insomnia or poor sleep quality can also be caused by a primary sleep disorder related to a medical condition. If the behavioral intervention is not working, or if your child has the warning signs mentioned below, then a sleep specialist consultation is a good idea.

A recent review highlighted that while most kids with ASD have behavioral sleep issues, which have been corroborated by objective measures such as actigraphy and polysomnography, at times children with ASD have true primary sleep disorders. The common primary sleep disorders include obstructive sleep apnea and periodic limb movements. Obstructive apnea is more likely in individuals who are overweight. Periodic limb movements occur often in children with restless legs syndrome; iron deficiency can contribute to restless legs syndrome and periodic limb movements. For children with ASD who have a limited diet, iron deficiency could be a possibility. For an individual child, the only definite way to identify a primary sleep problem is polysomnography.

Warning Signs of a Primary Sleep Disorder

Warning signs are not diagnostic, but they can help you decide whether your child might need a professional sleep evaluation. Watch for these signs in your child:

- Snores frequently even when not sick.

- Bedcovers frequently end up on the floor—even when it's cold.

- Is hanging half off the bed while sleeping (suggesting a lot of restless movement in sleep).

- Sleepwalks or has night terrors (wakes up screaming) more than once or twice.

- Can't wake up or resists getting up despite enough (apparent) sleep.

◈

Sleep Take-Home Points

- Blue screens interfere with sleep; limiting them helps sleep and creates more time for free play and exercise.

- Try to improve your child's sleep hygiene behaviorally first; that may do the trick for your child. Excellent self-help resources are available online from the National Sleep Foundation (*https://sleepfoundation.org*).

- If you are struggling to get your child's bedtime-related behavior into a positive place or suspect a sleep disorder, seek a professional evaluation.

Keep in mind that a healthy lifestyle is synergistic. It helps all children and helps physical and emotional health. If your child has ASD, your reduced margin for error makes improved exercise and sleep very attractive options to take advantage of. And each action step you decide to take is likely to boost the effects of the others. Exercise and sleep are a virtuous cycle—one promotes the other. And as you read the next chapter on what we know about food and ASD, keep in mind that a good diet also provides fuel for exercising. As you read through this book, think about what seems likely to help your child most, as well as what will be most practical for your family. The last chapter in the book will give you a chance to review all these ideas and choose the scientifically sound tools that will work for your child.

Establishing strong sleep habits and incorporating exercise into daily life are important life skills for everyone, whether you have a diagnosis of autism or not. Science increasingly tells us what we know from our own daily experience—that when we exercise regularly and are sufficiently rested we can manage challenges more readily, we engage with others more fluidly, we learn more effectively, and our mood is more stable. Although establishing these skills may be more challenging with your child with autism, putting effort into building this base of skills will have a lifelong impact for your child.

7

GASTROINTESTINAL AND FEEDING PROBLEMS, FOOD, AND DIET IN ASD

In 1943, when psychiatrist Leo Kanner published his groundbreaking paper describing autism, he noted that many of the children refused food, "vomited a great deal during the first year," or had "severe feeding difficulty from the beginning of life." He claimed these children were refusing food out of anxiety, as an attempt "to keep the outside world away," an interpretation that has not stood up to scientific scrutiny. But in the last 75 years, scientists have made great efforts to explore the food-related challenges of individuals with autism and have produced some key insights into how ASD and dietary issues are linked.

To begin with, systematic studies have confirmed what parents have reported: children with autism do indeed have gastrointestinal (GI) problems more frequently than other kids. According to data summaries and review studies published in 2018, four times more. The most common symptoms are constipation, diarrhea, and abdominal pain; other GI problems, such as reflux, don't seem to be elevated more than normal.

It's also increasingly clear that GI problems influence behavior, as you probably are well aware from your experience with your own child. Kids with GI discomfort are more irritable, can have trouble sleeping, and have more behavioral problems. This difficulty is understandably even more challenging for children who have less-well-developed speech and therefore can't communicate their discomfort. Children with intellectual limitations or delays may also experience more anxiety or confusion when they experience these symptoms. The box on pages 172–173 highlights some of the common signs and symptoms that may reflect GI discomfort. Interestingly, recent research has highlighted that autism-associated genes are involved in the development of both the central nervous system (the brain) and the enteric nervous system (the nerve system that controls the gut). This dovetails with rapidly emerging understanding that gut and brain are more heavily interconnected than previously thought—the so-called gut–brain axis. These systems share chemicals and pathways, such as the neurotransmitter serotonin, which has been implicated in autism, and also have multiple direct lines of communication.

FEEDING PROBLEMS IN AUTISM

Children with autism are also five times more likely than their peers to have what we call feeding problems ("picky eating"). These problems become especially worrisome when they affect a child's ability to get necessary nutrients or affect growth. Interestingly, though, a data summary of 881 children that found feeding problems more common in those with autism did not find significantly poorer growth or different intake of energy (carbohydrates and fats). Kids with ASD did have specific deficits (particularly reduced calcium and protein intake) that can have negative health effects, but we don't have a complete picture here since feeding problems haven't been studied as extensively as other health concerns in ASD. This might be because failure to thrive or declines in growth are more likely to trigger further evaluation per national health indicators.

> Children with autism are more likely to be picky eaters than their peers, but they don't seem to have growth problems or to take in fewer of the carbs and fats that supply energy.

If your child has feeding problems, it's important to bring them up with your child's pediatrician. Feeding problems can arise for many reasons, including difficulties with chewing and swallowing and sensitivities to different textures of food. Sometimes children

Signs and Symptoms of Gastrointestinal Problems to Watch For in Your Child with ASD

Even in typically developing kids, children and parents rarely agree on how much pain or discomfort the children are experiencing. Children often report that the gastrointestinal pain is much more severe than reported by parents. And research suggests that this discrepancy is much larger when a child is young and has few words to describe the symptoms. Therefore it can be important to watch for cues that your child is experiencing gastrointestinal pain and discomfort. A consensus report published in a 2010 supplement of *Pediatrics* (from the American Academy of Pediatrics) listed signs of GI discomfort, including these significant ones:

Vocal Cues

- Frequent clearing of throat, swallowing
- Sighing, whining, moaning, groaning, screaming
- Sobbing "for no reason at all"
- Stereotypic speech referencing pain or stomach (e.g., child says: "does your tummy hurt?" echoing a parental question)
- Direct verbalization of pain referencing the stomach

Motor Cues

- Facial grimacing
- Gritting teeth
- Wincing
- Constant eating/drinking/swallowing ("grazing" behavior)
- Mouthing behaviors: chewing on clothes (e.g., shirt sleeve cuff, neck of shirt)
- Application of pressure to abdomen (e.g., leaning abdomen against or over furniture, pressing hands into abdomen, rubbing abdomen)
- Finger tapping on throat
- Any unusual posturing (e.g., thrusting the jaw, twisting the neck, arching the back, positioning arms in odd ways, rotating the torso

or trunk in distorted ways, flinching or otherwise demonstrating sensitivity to being touched in the abdominal area)

- Agitation (e.g., pacing, jumping up and down)
- Unexplained increase in repetitive behaviors
- Self-injurious behaviors: biting, hits/slaps face, head banging, unexplained increase in self-injury
- Aggression: onset of, or increase in, aggressive behavior

Other Cues

- Sleep disturbances: difficulty getting to sleep, difficulty staying asleep
- Increased irritability
- Oppositional behavior in response to demands that typically do not result in oppositional behavior

While GI problems aren't the only cause of many of these signs and symptoms, they are one possible cause. If you see these cues and suspect gastrointestinal problems, seek a thorough evaluation from your child's physician. GI problems are treatable, and guidelines for how to treat GI problems in children with autism have been published.

develop fears of specific foods based on a past experience during which they gagged or experienced discomfort. Speech–language therapists, occupational therapists, and psychologists most commonly provide therapy for children with autism who have feeding problems. Because the cause of the problems is different for each child, the therapy program is individualized, focusing on increasing the diversity of foods the child will eat in some cases, providing swallowing lessons in others, and so forth. These therapy programs are typically very helpful.

Special Diets: Are They Helpful?

Despite the clear links between ASD and GI problems and picky eating, efforts to demonstrate that special diets can be helpful for most children with ASD so far are underwhelming. The most common idea has been to try restriction diets that limit gluten (found in wheat) or casein (found in dairy products). Results of these studies have been unconvincing thus far. We will discuss this in more detail later. Current research is investigating other supplements such as pre- and probiotics. While some initial studies are promising, studies aren't replicated or controlled well enough to inspire confidence in the results.

This picture may improve in years to come, but the challenges of conducting dietary clinical trials make progress slow. The fact that autism has so many different causes in different individuals (see Chapter 3) also limits the likelihood that a single dietary intervention will be effective for all. And it's been only recently that evidence has emerged about how the gut–brain axis contributes to autism. Yet, given the power of food and diet to influence feeling, mood, and behavior as well as gut health, it stands to reason that dietary interventions could help reduce challenging behaviors and increase prosocial communication. This is a ripe area for further research, and we'll provide whatever guidelines we can as we go through this chapter.

The Importance of Nutrition to Brain Development

As explained in Chapter 3, children's development is affected by both genes and environment, and appropriate fuel is critical for the development of all children. If your child has autism, however, nutrition is doubly important. So you'll want to stack the deck in your child's favor where diet is concerned.

What does that mean in today's world? It's not that easy to tease apart the appropriate path from the messages in the media regarding what foods to eat, what types of foods to avoid, or how much fat or carbohydrate is OK—all messages that seemingly flip-flop almost daily. But there are some key points that can help guide us.

One is that in the developed world many people are "overnourished"—or getting too many "empty calories" with lots of food but not enough nutrition. Another is that our food is often processed in ways that add nonfood chemicals (often to preserve the food or make it look more appetizing). These additives mean we can transport foods all over the world very cheaply without spoilage or loss, giving us a more balanced and palatable diet. But it also can come at a high cost to health that counteracts the benefits, as enumerated below. A third, and more positive, point is that nutrition is being shown to be a route to improved health and behavior that is often safe and therefore could be worth trying. In fact you can support your child's brain health and her physical health (preventing diet-related conditions like obesity and diabetes) through the same dietary measures. While a dietary treatment may not be effective at reducing symptoms for all children with autism, it may prove beneficial for some children. And for all children it can provide the foundation for healthy brain development and function.

FOOD AND THE BRAIN: WHAT SCIENCE TELLS US

We've long known about the relationship between the GI system and the brain. A clear example that has been known for decades is the inborn error of metabolism called phenylketonuria. PKU, as it is called, is a rare genetic disorder that results in the body's inability to metabolize phenylalanine, an amino acid common in many foods. Over time and exposure to the amino acid in the diet, phenylalanine builds up in the body and impacts brain functioning. This example is particularly relevant to autism because, prior to the identification of PKU, children with this genetic disorder were diagnosed with intellectual disability as well as autism. But when phenylalanine is eliminated from the diet, the amino acid doesn't build up in the brain and the child does not develop intellectual disability. Based on this observation, screening all newborns for PKU via a simple heel prick test began in earnest in the 1960s so that any who tested positive could receive dietary intervention starting at birth.

Now, thanks to new and better studies just in the past 5 years, we have scientific evidence for these additional modest but notable effects of diet:

- Food additives, food allergens, and food nutrients, particularly proper fat ratios, broadly influence attention, temperament, and behavior in typically developing children.
- Prenatal diet influences children's subsequent temperament and brain growth.
- Changing diet and omega-3 supplementation can sometimes

result in improvement in typically developing children or children with ADHD with certain symptoms that some children with autism also have, such as impulsivity, inattention, or emotional dysregulation.

How Food Communicates with the Brain: The Gut–Brain Axis

Fueling the interest in food's contribution to brain functioning has been the discovery of the microbiome (the microorganisms in the human body) and its relation to the communication channel called the gut–brain axis. We now know that the gut is connected to the brain via at least four major nerve and endocrine pathways. These pathways include brain chemicals, that is, neurotransmitters. This means that so-called brain chemicals are also in the gut, and that via the gut–brain axis the body's signals to the brain interact with the microbiome—including the community of microbes permanently living in the gut. There are many types of these microbes. One you may have heard of is called a probiotic. That discovery has spurred a recent craze for "probiotic supplements" among health-food enthusiasts—a "craze" not without some scientific support.

Scientists now study the human microbiome to understand its role in health and development. These microscopic organisms live all over our body, but most are in the digestive tract. A recent, striking discovery is that the human body contains more bacterial DNA than human DNA, and more bacterial than human cells! (It's also emerging that we have a lot of friendly viruses as well, but we know more about bacteria, so those are our focus.)

These friendly bacteria cover us and live throughout our body, helping us thrive. They and we have evolved together as a symbiotic co-organism over millions of years. Were it not for the bacteria, we would not be here. Were it not for us, they would not have taken anything like their current form. We cannot live without them, and they cannot live without us. They do everything from helping us digest food to sending signals to the rest of the body to guide energy allocation.

The gut and the brain "talk to each other" via specific nerve pathways that are only now being understood, including the vagus system, the enteric nervous system, the endocrine system (which is related to stress response as well as other functions), and the immune system. So, disruptions in part of the system can impact development and function in other parts of the system. To put it somewhat metaphorically, inflammation triggered in the gut can "travel" to the brain and affect brain function. That in turn can affect mood, attention, and behavior.

The most convincing research on the relevance of the gut to the brain and behavior has emerged in the past 10 years in animal experiments and

> *Via the gut–brain axis, inflammation in the gut can lead to disruptions in mood, behavior, and attention.*

mostly on animal behaviors that mimic human anxiety or mood. It seems almost certain that similar effects will hold for attention and other behaviors. While the microbiome is a current "hot topic," and therefore can be oversold, it nonetheless helps us understand just how vital diet and nutrition are to brain health.

It is important to note that brain growth and health doesn't depend on the microbiome alone. Brain activity relies heavily on the "macronutrients" of carbohydrates, proteins (amino acids), and fat, especially the long-chain fatty acids called omega-3s. It also relies on vitamin and mineral "micronutrients" such as iron, zinc, and calcium, which are crucial to neural transmission and brain health.

DIET DURING PREGNANCY AND EARLY CHILDHOOD: HOW FOOD MAY CHANGE THE RISK OF AUTISM AND WHAT YOU CAN DO ABOUT IT

Diet can affect brain growth directly by supplying (or not supplying) necessary nutrients. But nutrients also alter development by triggering epigenetic changes, both during pregnancy and after. These changes guide and support the growth of brain circuitry involved in learning, memory, motor and social development. However, the direct connection between diet-powered epigenetic changes and autism is still being studied and can at times be controversial. The field has many questions to answer:

- How much does a woman's diet during pregnancy affect the likelihood that her baby will end up having autism? Can her diet protect against other autism risk factors?

- What about the father's diet before conception? Does this affect risk?

- Is poor diet a direct cause of epigenetic changes that increase the risk of autism, or is it some other factor commonly associated with certain dietary habits that explains apparent correlations of diet with risk?

- What dietary measures can pregnant women take to compensate for other harms that might contribute to autism (and other health risks for the baby)?

- Can a child's diet in early life compensate for prenatal dietary (or other) risks and mitigate the symptoms of autism?

Obesity during Pregnancy

Some of the best evidence we have of a link between the dietary and metabolic health of a mother and her child's autism comes from studies of obesity during pregnancy. Obesity is epidemic in our society; it isn't due to diet alone, but most experts blame unhealthy diets for a significant part of the rise in obesity. Obesity in pregnancy is a difficult topic— many women have felt shamed and blamed by medical concerns about their weight in pregnancy. We don't want to promote such feelings; many overweight and obese women have healthy babies. Yet we also want to note the risks, which help provide clues to autism too. Obesity in pregnancy is associated with a child's increased risk for multiple health problems, including obesity, heart disease, asthma, psychiatric disorders, and neurodevelopmental disorders including autism. According to a recent summary of data from other studies, the risk of developing autism is about 1.5 times greater for a child with a mother who was obese during pregnancy than for a mother who had a normal body mass index.

Some of this risk can be reduced by careful tracking of weight gain during pregnancy. Other studies suggest that the risk increases for obese mothers who gain excess weight during pregnancy relative to their starting weight. Science also tells us that obesity prior to pregnancy increases the likelihood of maintaining an unhealthy diet in high-stress conditions, of which pregnancy is one. This means the risk of health problems in the baby, including autism, is compounded

Now a word of caution. Much of the evidence from human studies shows only a correlation—an association, not a direct cause—between maternal diet and autism and other health concerns. For example, women under more stress or economic hardship may more easily gain excess weight as well as have offspring with behavioral problems. Thus, we have to consider the possibility that the mother's obesity increased the risk of her child having autism, but it may have been that the stress she suffered was the key. Indeed, most obese moms will still not have children with autism. However, it seems likely that metabolic factors involving diet as well as obesity somehow combine with other factors to increase the chances a child will have autism.

To unravel causality, animal studies provide some insight. Animal studies in which scientists induce obesity in animals by feeding them high-fat diets (that is, a diet just like the typical American's) show a range of brain development effects in offspring when those animals become pregnant. These include increased susceptibility to behaviors that mimic anxiety and depression, impulsivity, and greater attentional deficits, as well as worse physical health. There is compelling evidence from these animal studies that these impacts are related to epigenetic changes that affect neurotransmitters such as serotonin, which is involved in attention and mood. While serotonin is associated with numerous behaviors, autism is on the list.

Unfortunately, we know little about the role of paternal diet or obesity, but we suspect, based on the existing animal literature on paternal effects from stress and chemical exposure, that it will prove to matter for child behavioral outcome too. One recent large study suggests that paternal obesity does increase the risk for autism in offspring, and possibly with an even larger effect than maternal obesity. Stay tuned to the research.

Nutrition and Brain Growth

Certain micro- and macronutrients also play a critical role in brain growth and the risk of autism. Micronutrients such as zinc, folate, vitamin B_{12}, vitamin A, and iron and macronutrients like omega-3s operate epigenetically and, during pregnancy, affect a baby's brain growth and also the risk for autism. For example, as mentioned in Chapter 3, when mothers take folic acid supplements during pregnancy, the risk of their babies' developing autism appears to decrease. However, some studies and recent reviews introduce a critical caution: *over*supplementing can increase risk for autism. Further, the benefit in relation to autism prevention may depend on the particular genotype or metabolic pattern of you and your child. Nonetheless, the balance of the evidence still indicates that it's important to follow medical guidelines for folate supplementation during pregnancy because it helps prevent severe problems like spina bifida.

The Good News: Fighting "Bad" Diet with "Good"

Women expecting a child can feel tremendous pressure to protect their unborn child from harm and try to control what is sometimes out of their control. They can also feel shame or guilt for what is out of their control, including their stress level, their body weight, and other factors. The good news, however, is that even if there are risk factors or genetic susceptibility, pregnant women can take actions that could confer some protection. The even better news is that most of these protective dietary factors are already recommended for everyone's overall health and also recommended by obstetricians for all pregnancies. Here are highlights and key action steps.

Upping Omega-3 Fatty Acids

A recent study in monkeys indicated that if monkey moms ate a typical American high-fat diet, the offspring had worse physical health and irritable temperaments. (They also demonstrated that these effects were related to epigenetic changes in the placenta and then in the baby monkeys' brains.) When the same mothers in the monkey study were fed sufficient doses of omega-3 fatty acids, their offspring were protected from the harmful effects of the diet. Because these experiments can randomly assign the animals to different conditions, they can rule out simple genetic effects on behavior as explaining the results. Other studies similar to this in rodents corroborate these results and suggest that sufficient maternal intake of "good fats" like omega-3 in pregnancy could prevent the epigenetic and health effects on offspring of the typical high-fat diet or of maternal overweight before or during pregnancy. Further research is needed to support these findings, but it can provide a plan of action to address the challenges with the American high-fat diet.

Reducing Saturated Fats and Trans Fats

Of course, in addition to increasing omega-3s, an even better approach is to reduce intake of the "bad fats." These are the fats that tend to contribute to obesity and other health problems. All of us should keep an eye on our consumption of them.

Taking Prenatal Vitamins

This is one of the first bits of advice an obstetrician typically gives expectant mothers: take your prenatal vitamins. As we just mentioned, the folic acid contained in these vitamins is very important here, despite some cautions about oversupplementation. Considering their positive effects on brain growth, those prenatal vitamins are like gold.

> Prenatal vitamins have such a positive effect on brain growth that they should be considered gold.

Diet in Your Child's Early Life

If you have been through a pregnancy after being very overweight or think you ate too much of a high-fat diet, it's not too late to try to counteract possible effects. The primary challenge in this realm for parents—for all of us—is simply finding healthy food for our children. Too often school lunches are loaded with added sugar or processed food with additives. At the grocery store, the lower-cost food is often the most processed and least healthy. Fresh and organic food, free of additives or pesticide residue, often costs more. While there are no silver bullets, in this regard there are two measures that most health organizations already recommend:

Breastfeeding

The safest and simplest way for young mothers to counteract negative influences during pregnancy is by breastfeeding. While not all women can manage this, it is really worth trying to make it work. (If you are having trouble with breastfeeding, counselors can sometimes suggest behavioral approaches that will make it go easier.) If you can possibly do it, standard recommendations suggest you breastfeed for at least 6 months. However, the American Academy of Pediatrics recommends that you breastfeed for 12 months (introducing other foods after 6 months of age as a complement to, but not a replacement for, breast milk). In the small number of studies done to date, a connection was found between more breastfeeding and lower risk of autism and autism symptoms, but we don't know if that is a causal effect or how reliable it is—some literature suggests that there is no relationship. However, the World Health Organization (WHO) shows that breastfed babies have a more gradual, healthy weight gain than formula-fed babies, and WHO encourages breastfeeding as late as 24 months of age. So, it's a good idea in general, and there's an outside chance it adds to your child's protection against autism risk.

Omega-3 Supplements

Your child's diet may be able to overcome negative epigenetic effects of prenatal diet, at least in part, by once again supplementing with omega-3. Given omega-3s' contribution to supporting brain health and addressing epigenetic changes, it is promising. However, we have to note that there is very limited evidence to suggest that this will have a specific effect on preventing or reducing autism symptoms. Systematic reviews of randomized clinical trials suggest that omega-3 supplementation as an intervention for autism is not effective. Given the limited literature, it may be that future, larger studies will overturn that preliminary conclusion. For now, omega-3s are a good idea in general but not a remedy for autism. That said, happily, breast milk delivers a lot of omega-3s to babies, and adverse effects associated with omega-3 supplementation appear to be minimal.

✦

Dietary Action Steps for Pregnancy
and Early Life That Are Safe and Might Help

- *If you are pregnant or planning to get pregnant:*
  - Do your best to keep your weight gain within the range recommended by your doctor.

- Increase your intake of omega-3s through diet or supplements, take prenatal vitamins, and reduce saturated and trans fats (under supervision of your doctor).
- *If you think risk is high that your infant will have autism:*
  - Consider breastfeeding (or feeding pumped breast milk) for the first 12 months.
  - Consider omega-3 supplementation.

DIETARY INTERVENTIONS FOR CHILDREN WITH AUTISM

Because brain development continues into young adulthood, it's never too late to "feed" your child's brain healthful nutrients. And although we have limited evidence that doing so can directly improve the symptoms of autism, there are some commonsense approaches that stack the deck in your favor by providing an optimal environment for your child to benefit from those treatments and interventions that do work. So, if your child has been diagnosed with autism or is showing some of the signs, it's prudent to look at his diet to make sure you've covered all the bases.

Doing so, however, can be challenging since you will encounter a lot of different proposed interventions, which run the gamut from not well supported but with limited adverse effects to very poorly supported and even dangerous. Among the various proposals that you are likely to encounter are:

- Omega-3 fatty acid supplements
- Nutrient/vitamin supplements (e.g., zinc or vitamin B_{12})
- The gluten-free, casein-free (GFCF) diet
- Other restriction or elimination diets (e.g., "ketogenic diet")
- Avoiding specific additives (such as food coloring or sugar)

The scientific literature regarding dietary interventions for autism is still emerging, and as of the writing of this book most studies have failed to show that dietary changes have positive effects on autism symptoms. This is due partly to a lack of well-designed studies and partly to the fact that autism is so heterogeneous that it's difficult to find particular interventions that benefit whole groups of children with autism. Note, however, that this does not rule out the possibility that some individuals with autism will benefit from a certain intervention.

An updated recent systematic review of nutritional and dietary interventions for autism that took place between 2010 and 2016 included studies on omega-3 supplementation, GFCF diets, digestive enzymes (proteolytic enzyme supplements, digestive enzyme supplements), and methyl B_{12} supplementation. This review drew the same conclusions as the previous review based on all studies between 2000 and 2010. The evidence to date does not show that nutritional supplements or the GFCF diet improve autism symptoms or gastrointestinal complaints. A similar review of randomized controlled trials published in 2017 focused solely on supplementation and reached the same conclusion. One key finding from these reviews, however, is that few adverse effects are associated with these dietary and nutritional interventions.

What, Then, Are Parents to Do?

Let's start with common sense: If a child is overweight, eating empty calories, or not getting good nourishment, she will be more tired, listless, and unmotivated, won't feel good, and won't feel like focusing on anything that may be challenging (such as attending to the social world in the case of autism). You likely have seen this yourself in your own children or others. If your child is eating too much junk food—processed, filled with additives, and containing sugar (in all its myriad forms)—her energy is likely to be inconsistent and her mood less mellow. These effects alone can in turn make self-regulation challenging. So, step one is to maintain a healthy, balanced diet. Easier said than done when your child's food preferences are restricted to only white foods, or only crunchy foods, or foods without particular smells. (We'll address this later in this chapter.)

Beyond this broad dietary prescription, we follow the same rules stated in Chapter 6: If an intervention makes sense and is safe, we require less evidence to accept it than if it doesn't pass the gut check (no pun intended) or is risky. Let's look at the commonly proposed interventions listed above.

- *Omega-3s: Not effective in trials to date for ASD symptoms, but relatively safe and easy and may help secondary problems like inattention or mood.* Omega-3s are found in most kinds of fish, eggs, olive oil, avocados, and other foods. When we were evolving, our diet probably included a lot more omega-3 fatty acid foods, so the ratio between different kinds of fat in our blood (omega-3, omega-6, and others) was a lot different than it is today. Over the last hundred years, at least in the West, the average diet has shifted toward a lot fewer of the foods that contain omega-3s. An easy solution, then—if your child likes them—would be to increase omega-3 consumption by serving more of the foods that contain them. As mentioned above, the literature does not suggest that omega-3 supplementation will improve autism symptoms, but because of the positive impacts of omega-3 on brain development, it could still be of great value, because it might mean your child can get by with less medication or respond more effectively to treatments. For children, the risks of omega-3 supplementation are that fish-oil tablets can cause stomach upset, headache, insomnia, temporary diarrhea, or elevated blood readings of certain fats. One trial suggested about 5% of children experience one or more of these side effects. To prevent these effects, give the tablets with food and lower the dose if digestion problems occur. The good news is that there is almost no risk to adding more of these fats to your child's diet other than stomach upset or diarrhea at very high doses.

- *Nutrient/vitamin supplementation: Use only if your child is deficient.* Iron and zinc are crucial to cell signaling and efficient nervous system functioning. Your child needs the right amount. Although animal studies show that a lack of these nutrients can lead to epigenetic effects on development, human studies have failed to show that blindly giving iron or zinc supplements to all children with autism helps. Further, too much iron or zinc is dangerous. If your child has autism or symptoms associated with low nutrient levels (such as restless legs syndrome, which is associated with iron deficiency) and if he is not eating nutritious foods, it may make sense to get his blood levels checked. A surprising number of children have low iron levels, especially during periods of rapid growth. If blood levels indicate a deficiency, it makes sense to supplement, but only in collaboration with your doctor. Otherwise, proceed with caution or avoid supplements, as overdosing can be dangerous.

Vitamin D is not as risky, but the story is much the same. Many children, particularly in northern latitudes, including the northern third of the United States, have low vitamin D. But even in sunny climates, children are often indoors and don't get enough sunlight. It can make sense to get your child's vitamin D blood levels checked and supplement if necessary, but there's no evidence that supplementing beyond those levels will improve symptoms of autism.

For most other single-nutrient supplements either research has shown no impact or we don't have enough data to draw conclusions regarding autism. So don't supplement with zinc, vitamin D, iron, calcium, or other single supplements outside of a measured deficiency.

 • *The GFCF diet: Not shown to be effective for ASD and difficult to follow, but relatively safe.* The GFCF diet, the most commonly used dietary intervention for autism, removes food and drinks that contain gluten (a protein in wheat, barley, and rye) and casein (a protein in milk and dairy products) and was originally proposed as a treatment for autism based on the hypothesis that (1) individuals with autism are unable to break down these proteins and have a leaky gut, which absorbs peptides associated with this failure to break down the proteins; (2) this process leads to pain and associated behavioral challenges; (3) these peptides travel into the central nervous system through the leaky gut and bind to opioid receptors; and (4) this results in changes in brain development and autism-related symptoms. A number of scientific studies of the GFCF diet have been conducted, and recent systematic reviews conclude that there is little evidence that the diet improves autism symptoms. Of the four randomized trials to date, the two studies that are well designed and controlled demonstrate no effectiveness, while the other two studies, which are not as well controlled and likely influenced by the perspective of the scientists and the parent participants, find support for the diet. The diet requires a lot of effort to maintain, although there are few side effects. Four small studies simply do not provide enough data to either support or refute the use of the GFCF diet.

 • *The ketogenic diet: Not effective for ASD symptoms and difficult to implement, with potential side effects.* The ketogenic diet has gained recognition as an effective treatment for individuals with particular genetic disorders and, more broadly, for epilepsy (which has as

How Do You Know a Study of Diet and Autism Is Reliable?

The following are the major considerations for a scientific design.

1. Are the measures valid—for example, was autism carefully defined? Was diet measured carefully? A clinic study may have far better measurement than a national survey.

2. How large and generalizable is the sample? For example, a study of children referred to a clinic may be biased because only children with insurance and multiple problems come in for care. A national survey may have far better generalizability than a clinic study.

3. Is the study causal or correlational? As we've explained, correlation is not causation. Different studies merit different levels of confidence.

a. A cross-sectional, correlational study observes that children who have autism also have some other characteristics, like low blood levels of vitamin D. But this does not prove that one caused the other. Kids with autism might stay indoors more and thus have less vitamin D, or a third factor not measured, such as living in a region with a dark climate or limited health care, might explain both points.

b. A prospective study controls for what came first. Children are enrolled before they have autism or an exposure, and the outcomes are looked at. For example, children might be enrolled at birth and their existing lead level measured. Then subsequent lead exposure is measured, and after that, autism outcome. Studies of this type yield stronger results than simple cross-sectional studies.

c. "Natural experiments" provide even more hints about causation. For example, researchers can see whether autism is more likely to occur after smoking by surrogate mothers who are not genetically related to the child.

d. As described in Chapter 1, the gold standard for causality is the double-blind, randomized controlled trial. By randomly assigning participants to different treatments, such as an experimental dietary supplement or an identical-looking and -tasting food (with different ingredients), with the participants (and the experimental observers) unaware of their treatment group, differences in outcomes can be attributed to the dietary intervention and not something else.

many different causes as autism). The diet includes high-fat foods with protein to ensure growth, but significantly limited carbohydrate intake. The result is that the body uses fat primarily as a fuel source. Given the success of the diet in other populations, it has become of interest to the autism community. To date two studies have examined this dietary intervention in autism. The first study reported symptom reduction for children with autism who were treated with the diet, but, importantly, the study was not a trial (no control group or randomization or blinding). The second study was a case report of a single individual receiving the diet with a report of positive outcomes. So there is currently no evidence for the effectiveness of this treatment, the diet itself can be difficult to establish, and side effects can be considerable, given the significant modifications to the diet.

- *Avoiding specific additives (artificial food colors or dyes, etc.): Limited evidence that additives contribute to ASD symptoms, but easy to avoid with a healthy diet.* The degree of evidence linking additives to health or behavioral reactions is variable, and there are many additives in our food today. The following are some of the more common:
  - Artificial colors
  - Artificial flavors and flavor enhancers (monosodium glutamate [MSG]
  - or monopotassium glutamate)
  - Artificial sweeteners (aspartame, acesulfame K, neotame, saccharin, sucralose)
  - Preservatives and stabilizers (sodium benzoate, butylated hydroxyanisole [BHA], butylated hydroxytoluene [BHT], carrageenan)
  - Protein extenders (for example, hydrolyzed, textured, or modified protein)

There is some evidence to suggest that artificial food dyes and/or preservatives impact behaviors related to autism, but the evidence is far from convincing. The good news is that you can avoid or reduce food additives simply by focusing on nonprocessed, nutrient-dense foods (fresh produce, fresh meat, whole grain bread and pasta). A couple of easy hints:

- Read labels, and if you see ingredients that you're not familiar with, don't have in your kitchen, or would not use in your own cooking, don't buy the food.

- Find fresh food by shopping the outside aisles of the super-market.

DEALING WITH PICKY EATING

Scientific reports reflect what parents report: for many individuals with autism, eating behavior is significantly restricted by food category and by texture and there is a much higher rate of food refusal than in typically developing children. Interestingly, though, one study found that family food preferences influence food selection more than the diagnosis of autism does. That is, the fewer food items a family eats, the fewer food items the children with autism ate. So while these children still had a more limited palate than typically developing children, the more types of food the parents ate, the more types of food the children with autism ate.

One of the most pernicious myths is that children who will not eat healthy food have to be given "something" they will eat. Science does not bear this out. What experiments show is that if all the choices given to children are healthy, children will choose one of the options and eat it. Example: Snacks may be carrots, apple slices, nuts, or cheese. Drink choices can be water or milk (no sugary drink). A child may complain the first day the "new options" come into effect, but ultimately the child will eat—he will not starve himself. You can just matter-of-factly provide the available options. You can't rely on children's "instinct" for choosing healthy food or getting the nutrients they need when unhealthy food is available. Their bodies are smart but evolved before processed food did. Their instincts don't know how to filter healthy from unhealthy food if it is tasty. Even mice become malnourished when offered sugary along with healthy food. The keys:

- Provide choices.
- Provide only healthy choices.
- If all the choices are healthy, then kids can pretty much eat what they want.

✦

Action Steps for Managing GI and Feeding Problems and Improving Diet

You've heard all this before, but now your understanding of the gut–brain axis may underscore the importance of focusing on diet in autism. It is clear that gastrointestinal problems exist more frequently for individuals with autism, and while it's unclear specifically how that relates to dietary interventions, improving diet with commonsense approaches helps brain development and the gastrointestinal system:

1. Minimize fast food: Cook at home (and keep it simple to avoid driving yourself crazy) or get good-quality prepared meals elsewhere most days.
2. Provide plenty of fresh fruits and vegetables.
3. Minimize processed food.
   a. Use whole grains instead of processed or refined grains.
   b. Minimize junk food, soda, or juices that include any type of sugar in the label.
4. If your child has ongoing GI or feeding issues, be sure to discuss these with your child's pediatrician because these problems can significantly influence your child's growth and nutrition.

The Specifics

- *Stay fresh.* Shift your family to more fresh fruits and vegetables; minimize boxed and packaged food products.

- *Shop outside.* Shop the outside aisles of the store to avoid processed food.

- *Go organic.* To avoid pesticide residue, supplements, and additives, buy organic foods.

- *Sardines are your friend.* Eat plenty of cold-water fish to get omega-3 fatty acids or choose a high-quality purified (USP-labeled) fish oil supplement with 1–2 grams of omega-3, at least half EPA. (Unfortunately, scientific-sounding claims for various omega-3-type products are rife on the Internet; ask your health-food store buyer to suggest a high-quality product.)

- *Monitor allergens.* Avoid allergenic foods if your child shows any reactions.

- *Check blood levels.* Ask your doctor to check your child's blood levels of iron, zinc, vitamin D, or other minerals as well as omega-3s during routine physicals.

- *Limit sugar.* Although not specific to autism, sugar is a major health risk. Sharply limit added sugar and sugary drinks.

- *No caffeine.* Eliminate caffeine for preadolescent or growing children.

- *Don't sweat the rest.* Ignore the maze of other dietary suggestions for autism.

The good news here is that the upshot—to get your family on a healthy diet—is a good idea even if you aren't sure it will help with autism. We don't need autism research to carry out the suggestions here; they all make good health sense for everyone. What's new is the recognition that these foundations can support and prepare your child to benefit most from treatments that work.

Simply by moving your family to a healthy diet of fresh foods prepared (as much as possible) and eaten at home, cutting out sugary drinks and processed food, and eating organic fruits and vegetables (to avoid pesticide residues and because they are usually fresher), you can achieve a great deal. This approach will increase nutrient value, avoid additives like food coloring, and reduce total sugar intake for your child. If you include plenty of cold-water fish, your child will get ample omega-3 fatty acids as well. The principal additions that are autism specific are to make sure to get the omega-3 fatty acids and have your doctor check your child's blood levels of iron, zinc, and vitamin D if there is any doubt about those nutrients.

8

TECHNOLOGY AND ASD

Latest Findings on the Peril and the Promise

Electricity, telephones, televisions, home computers, smartphones. Technological advances in the past 150 years have radically changed all aspects of life from work to parenting, and electronic and social media now play a major role in children's lives. By age 4, a majority of children are multitasking electronically.

Parents have always wondered about the role of technology in their children's lives: "Does playing that video game lead to violence?" "Is it OK to let my child watch TV every night?" To think that the phone that is tucked into your pocket today is more powerful than the room-sized computers that helped land Neil Armstrong on the moon speaks to how quickly technology is changing and the scope and reach of everyday technology today. Perhaps not surprisingly, the Internet is rife with speculation about the influences of social media and technology on children with ASD, both good and bad. Parents understandably have many questions about the role of technology in their children's lives.

While advances in technology offer promise of novel diagnostic approaches and treatments for autism, bona fide social interaction will always be the best way of engaging children and helping them grow and learn. Technology might offer a way of augmenting treatment, but it cannot substitute for real interactions with other people. What does the science say about technology and autism? In this chapter we'll sift through a burgeoning scientific literature to separate fact from hype or unwarranted concern, highlight what we know about technology-related autism treatments, and review what we know about screen time and autism. We will aim to address key questions that you may have, such as "How much screen time is too much screen time?" "Will video games make my child inattentive or less socially adept?" or "Are there technological tools to help treat my child's autism?" Let's start by looking at both the benefits and downsides of technology.

TECHNOLOGY: OPPORTUNITY OR RISK FOR AUTISM?

The informational, educational, and therapeutic potential of today's computer electronics, crammed into devices that fit into our pockets, or on our wrists, or even on our eyeglasses, is mind-boggling. And the range and scope of what the various gadgets and tools can do is constantly evolving with new hardware, software, and social media platforms continually emerging. It's hard to keep up with what it all does, for good or ill. What do you need to know about how technology interacts with your child on the spectrum?

There's no doubt that technology can impact behaviors associated with autism, as we'll discuss later in the chapter. But to start with, it's important to keep in mind that most devices have blue-light screens that can interfere with melatonin production and sleep, as described in Chapter 6.

In addition, most devices (and even some watches) provide children with access to the Internet, where they can find everything from social networking sites to search engines, shopping pages, and video offerings. They can communicate, share photos and other files, and chat. On the positive side, children get access to extraordinary amounts of information and opportunities to learn and be educated *if* they can manage it all and learn how to navigate the information. On the negative side, that's a big "if" for most kids, and Internet access comes with some additional risks that are common concerns of parents, hyped by media and of varying risk level:

- Distracting, attention-grabbing information that may affect attention and focus
- Violent content that can be distracting or overstimulating, or inspire harmful actions

- Pornographic, explicit, or disturbing sexual content beyond one's maturity level
- Disclosure of personal information for public viewing
- Sexual predators
- Online bullying and harassment
- Ideological extremists (such as terrorist groups)
- Comment boards filled with nasty, hostile, or demeaning exchanges
- Social isolation and reduced opportunities for face-to-face interaction

To make parents' worries more complicated, websites, games, and interactive media are psychologically sophisticated, capitalizing on some of the most powerful teaching technologies ever developed and appealing to unconscious needs. By design, their frequent yet unpredictable feedback to the user makes them inherently rewarding and habit forming. This feature can be powerful for inspiring engaged learning. However, these tools, which can have true educational and entertainment value (and truly can give parents a much-needed break), also have a dark side when it comes to children's healthy development of brain functioning, self-control, prosocial behavior, social skills, and attention. On top of that, besides interfering with sleep quality, media use can compete with exercise, free play, and homework!

So, what does the science tell us?

What Does the Science Tell Us about Media Use and Autism?

Does too much screen use hurt social development in a way that makes ASD worse? One might think this is an easy question to answer, but the literature on this is mixed. While a handful of studies based on smaller samples and surveys suggest that children with autism watch TV earlier and spend more time using screens than their peers, a large study across the United States suggests that there are no differences in screen-time exposure for children with autism and their peers. However, research has also suggested that children with autism who are using electronic media are doing so without parent or caregiver interaction. That is, they're watching TV or using other media, like YouTube or video games, on their own. So for them, screen time and television viewing are a less social experience than for other children who are watching with family. Another study found that rates of technology use varied by specific types of technology. For example, teens with ASD had higher rates of electronic media use, as well as of non–social media use, relative to peers. While the overall findings regarding media use and autism are complex, it is safe to conclude that media use appears to be different for children with autism than for their peers. These findings don't mean that electronic media use is causing autism; rather, they suggest that children with autism use electronic media differently.

> For children with autism, screen time is often a solitary pursuit, and is less socially oriented than for other kids.

Does Electronic Media Exposure Cause Autism?

Strictly speaking, the short answer is no. As we discussed earlier in this book, autism arises from a combination of multiple genetic and environmental risk factors that influence brain development during prenatal and early postnatal life. Thus, electronic media is likely not a significant causal factor. However, that doesn't mean it's unimportant—media use can affect language, social, and emotional development and so can compound the challenges of a child who has ASD.

Let's explore the question of a causal connection between ASD and electronic media use a bit more. The theory that autism is caused by television exposure has been proposed, and one empirical paper also makes this claim. However, these claims are all based on correlational data—the observation of children with ASD spending more time or different kinds of time on screens. Remember, correlation is not causation. While it is possible that too much screen time takes away from spending time with other people and thereby influences social development, it is also possible that because infants and children with ASD have difficulty with social interaction, they may be more attracted to screen use. For example, research in typically developing children finds that infants who are more active and fussy and who have sleep or feeding problems are exposed to more TV. We know that infants who develop ASD are often temperamentally different from infants who don't develop ASD and have higher rates of sleeping and feeding problems (see Chapters 6 and 7). Given that relationship, infants who go on to receive a diagnosis of autism may end up being exposed to TV more than their peers.

One of the papers positing that TV may be a cause of autism reported a correlation between the rise of autism prevalence and growth in access to cable television over roughly two decades in California and Pennsylvania, from 1972 to 1989. While they found a rise in both autism rates and cable TV access, they found that the rise in autism was more rapid in counties where more homes had access to cable TV. Further, based on reports that higher levels of precipitation are associated with more TV viewing in all children, they looked at the correlation between rates of autism and rainfall across counties in Washington, Oregon, and California and found higher rates of autism in counties with more rainfall. Putting those findings together, they concluded that TV exposure may play a causal role in autism. While that is one interpretation, this is purely circumstantial evidence. Countless explanations for this correlation are possible. For example, counties with greater access to cable TV may also have greater access to clinical services and greater diagnostic awareness, resulting in higher autism rates. Counties with greater rainfall may have larger population concentrations (and therefore services and awareness), which will also increase autism rates. The preponderance of research points to genetics interacting with early environmental experience (in utero). If screen exposure plays a role in worsening ASD, the effect is likely very slight. To date, we have no strong evidence that it does or doesn't.

Does Screen Time Impact Your Child's Autism Symptoms?

The broader question of social–emotional and language development is a little more complex because of the wide range of challenges an individual with autism may have and the many effects electronic media use can have on social, emotional, language, and cognitive development. Let's look at the issues that are most difficult to evaluate first.

Social Abilities

How might media use impact social skills? We know that, particularly for the youngest children, language learning depends on language interchange with caregivers. So the fact that use of screens takes time away from social interactions means excessive exposure can start to interfere with the pace of early language development (as well as preliteracy learning, according to some studies). We know in fact that excessive TV exposure in early child development is associated with social–emotional delays in typical children and that there's evidence of a causal connection since observational studies show that background TV, for example, disrupts social interactions between children and caregivers. Thus, the relationship between poorer social–emotional functioning and increased television viewing is thought to be the result of fewer parent–child interactions and overall poorer family functioning generally, as well as exposure to inappropriate adult content.

The picture for adolescents is, once again, more complex. Some large-scale studies report that increased screen time is correlated with poor attachment and relationships, while other large-scale studies report no relationship. The key point here is that in the absence of clear directives from the literature regarding media use and autism, we can apply what we know from the literature in typically developing children. The take-home message is that attending to the social world will certainly provide more opportunities for your child with autism to develop and practice social skills than watching TV or using an iPad or smartphone.

That said, you may have heard that some iPad and other electronic programs have educational value. This can be true—but only if you as caregiver are interacting with the child and the media. Very young children learn language far better when they hear it from caregivers than when exposed to it on media. Parent amplification of what's on the media, however, is beneficial with the right content—that is, content focused on promoting prosocial behavior and learning skills. (For further recommendations on optimizing the use of media by your child with ASD, see the box on pages 198–199.)

> When in doubt about media use, make sure that media use involves a social element.

Language

Research does make some connections between screen time and language development, but as with social development, the relationship is complex. Reviews of many studies that have examined the impact of media

Managing Media Time

The American Academy of Pediatrics lists the following guidelines regarding reasonable amounts of media time:

- *For children under 18 months old:* Avoid screen media use except for video chatting. Activities should focus on hands-on, interactive activities with others.

- *For children between 18 and 24 months old:* If digital media is introduced at this age, it should be high-quality programming, and parents should watch it with their children to help promote understanding of what is being watched. Most time should be spent engaging in interactive activities with others.

- *For children between 2 and 5 years old:* Screen use should be limited to 1 hour per day of high-quality programs that are also watched by the parents to promote understanding of what is being watched.

- *For children 6 years of age and older (including adolescents):* Consistent limits should be placed on the types of media and time spent using media. Parents should make sure media does not interfere with behaviors critical to health, such as sleep, family meals, physical activity, and "unplugged" downtime. Screen-free times (bedtime, mealtime) and screen-free locations (bedroom, dinner table) should be established.

- *For children of all ages:* Media should be viewed alongside children to help them learn from what they are doing, seeing, and saying online. Essentially, parents should be a "media mentor" to help guide media use.

For children with autism we want to make sure that the limits are on the lower end of the range so that more opportunities for practice of social interactions are promoted.

The following recommendations can be useful for addressing some of the challenges that arise with use of screen media by children with autism:

1. To manage increased use of media and difficulties disengaging from media:

   - Use auto timers on devices so that the device shuts off automatically after the decided time limit has been exceeded.

- Use transition reminders.
- Use consistent daily times.

2. To incorporate developmental delays:
   - Follow media guidelines that are consistent with your child's mental age, not his chronological age.

3. To address reduced time spent engaging in physical activity or with friends:
   - Use media time as a reward for engaging in physical activity or spending time in social activities.
   - Use apps or programs that encourage physical fitness and social interaction.

4. To avoid using media time as a "pacifier":
   - Given that the use of media time as a pacifier will actually increase the likelihood of tantrums, be sure to make only limited use of media as a reward for good behavior.
   - Do not use media time to reduce tantrums or challenging behaviors in the moment. Use other coping strategies to deescalate challenging behaviors.

5. To address limited understanding of sexuality and violence:
   - Provide education about the consequences of sexual and violent behavior.
   - Monitor screen time closely to attend to cyberbullying, inappropriate comments, or potential exploitation.

on cognitive and language development suggest that the effect of media depends on three factors: (1) the age of the child, (2) the type of programming (educational programming versus noneducational), and (3) the social context in which the media viewing occurs. Research suggests that for very young children (less than 2 years old), television viewing mostly has a negative impact, especially for language development and executive function skills. For preschool-age children, the impact of television viewing depends on the content of the media. Several studies have found that educational programs such as *Sesame Street* actually have a positive influence on language and cognitive skill development. There haven't been a lot of studies on the impact of television on older children. However, some studies have shown that educational computer programs can promote some academic skills.

A key factor is whether your child is watching television or playing games by herself or with others. Noneducational programs studied usually include computer games, which can be a social activity. Recent research suggests that media use can help promote language development when used in conjunction with a caregiver. The key here is caregiver–child interaction, which is the richest environment for language learning. For your child with autism, then, it's wise to limit media and screen use as well as solo electronic media use so that face-to-face social interactions can scaffold language as well as social development.

Sleep

Many studies have examined the impact of digital media use on sleep in children, most conducted with children with typical development. Importantly, since we know that autism brings sleep problems (see Chapter 6), these findings likely apply to children with autism as well. The majority of studies in typically developing children find that greater use of digital screen-based media is associated with more sleep problems, including a delay in the time the child or adolescent falls asleep and how long the child sleeps.

Getting ample sleep is critical to many aspects of health and well-being. Excessive consumption of digital media apparently contributes to sleep problems by displacing the time a child should be sleeping with screen time, overstimulating the child before bedtime, making it harder to fall asleep, and reducing the total time the child is sleeping. In addition, the light emitted from devices has been found to affect circadian rhythm (the body's "biological clock,"

> *Since screen time can displace sleep time—or lead to overstimulation—it's wise to limit screen time to promote good sleep hygiene, particularly before bed.*

which regulates when we feel sleepy vs. alert), as well as sleep itself (e.g., how deep the sleep is). For all of these reasons, you should take care that use of digital media near bedtime is not contributing to or worsening your child's sleep difficulties.

Attention

As discussed earlier in this book, many children with autism struggle with symptoms like inattention, hyperactivity, and impulsivity or have a diagnosis of ADHD in addition to their autism diagnosis. Research on media use in ADHD has suggested that screen time has a small but significant impact on ADHD symptoms, specifically inattention. In 2015, scientists put together the first meta-analysis of screen media use and ADHD that was based on enough studies to be authoritative. They found that there is in fact an overall association between more screen media use and more symptoms of ADHD—including a few experimental studies that support a causal linkage. As you might suspect, this is particularly the case for inattention, rather than hyperactivity or impulsivity. However, this association is quite small—certainly smaller than the effect of media on aggression, and also smaller than most other risk factors for ADHD. Whether this average effect masks greater effects for some children is unknown, and what might cause the association is unclear. Do the screens directly disrupt attention development? Or do they simply prevent children from the hands-on engagement with people and things they need to grow their brain fully, and thus indirectly interfere with development?

Aggression

Some children with autism display aggressive behavior. Often the aggression is reactionary, tied to attempts to escape from a situation or task, or linked to pain or discomfort for individuals who have limited verbal means of communicating needs and wishes. While the literature regarding media use, particularly violent video games, and aggression is clear, it's less clear how that interfaces with the types of aggression associated with autism.

Scientists have known for quite a long time that unrestricted TV and video games hurt children due to the violence they contain. An hour a day of unrestricted commercial television will mean a child witnesses, in one week, dozens of extreme violent acts (murders, assaults, rape). This is true in cartoons as well as dramas. Art does not "reflect life" here; screen media show a lot more violence than actually exists in the world, giving children a distorted understanding of the social world.

The science shows that this exposure to screen violence causes more aggressive acting-out behavior both in the short term and over the life-span. This is one of the most well-established findings in the field of psychology—and one of the least well known. More than a decade ago, the Association for Psychological Science published an authoritative summary in its publication *Psychological Science in the Public Interest.* The scientific evidence here is conclusive, with a large, varied set of hundreds of observational and experimental studies. Comprehensive literature reviews of hundreds of studies have produced the same picture: TV and game violence increases aggression in children.

> One of the most well-established findings in psychology is that exposure to screen violence causes more aggressive behavior in the short and long term.

How could this exposure impact your child with autism? During day-to-day life we rely on automatic routines and scripts to help govern our behavior to make life easier and more fluid. For example, we often don't even think about introducing ourselves and extending our hand to shake when meeting someone new. We rely on our "meeting someone" script so that we aren't using so much brain power to navigate that situation. We exert mental control in situations where we need to override these scripts. Building on the above greeting example, I (Bernier) often greet my patients and their caregivers in the waiting room with a handshake, but recently a mother of a patient was not allowed to touch other men because of her religious beliefs. After learning this, I wished to remain respectful of this and so I had to exert mental control to override my handshake greeting script when approaching her in the lobby. Relevant to this discussion is that our scripts are based on our experience and what we are exposed to in the media. Media violence primes the automatic parts of our psyche with scripts, routines, and schemas that involve aggressive behavior. In the heat of the moment, during times when mental control is most needed, people who watch more media violence are more prone to activate these automatic aggressive scripts. Not all children are affected equally; some are practically immune to these media effects. However, some children with autism—say, the children with autism who also struggle with impulsivity—may rely on automatic scripts that have been influenced by this violent media exposure, increasing the likelihood that aggressive behavior will be the selected automatic script when the child is upset or during a tantrum.

Internet Gaming Addiction

Internet gaming addiction, as defined by the WHO, is gaming behavior that is difficult to control, impacts participation in other activities, continues despite negative consequences, and impacts personal, family, social, educational, or occupational functioning. In DSM-5, a new disorder called "Internet gaming disorder" was added to the section on "conditions needing further research." The DSM-5 definition is similar to the WHO definition, but it includes additional possible symptoms, such as making unsuccessful attempts to stop playing, using deception to hide playing, or playing to escape negative mood states. As with the WHO definition, the combination of symptoms must be severe enough to cause interference in life activities. It is important to note that these criteria overlap heavily with the criteria for gambling addiction and partially with those for substance use disorders.

Specific diagnostic criteria have been developed in response to the exploding clinical demand for help with youth struggling with addictive or addiction-like behavior associated with video gaming. Not surprisingly, the gaming manufacturers have objected to the labeling of this pattern of behavior, but scholars have raised doubts too, stating that this labeling is premature. Despite these concerns, the overall consensus is that gaming addiction is a serious clinical problem because of the associated social isolation, negative impact on sleep, reduced physical activity and dietary problems, decreased psychological well-being, interference with academics or job, and interpersonal conflicts.

The potential for addiction to online gaming to be a problem has been noted for children with ADHD for over a decade but has really come into focus in the last 5 years. For children with autism it's only been a recent concern, and there is now preliminary research to suggest that Internet addiction is more common among children with autism than among their peers. It makes sense given the increased atypical media use for children with autism reported in the literature. Additionally, we often hear reports of individuals with autism having difficulty transitioning from media use to other activities. Also, the restricted and repetitive interests and behaviors that are part of the diagnostic criteria for autism make the focus on video games and video game content particularly compelling for individuals with autism.

The existing literature suggests that risk factors include being male, being a teenager, and

> Research shows that Internet addiction is more common among children and teens on the spectrum, particularly teenage boys who have trouble controlling their impulses.

struggling with impulsivity. This is a behavior that will be important to monitor for your child with autism. We don't currently have any randomized controlled studies to help us determine effective treatments, but the best intervention is likely to be a cognitive-behavioral therapy (CBT) approach. The downside here is that the individual is going to have to be willing to address the problem. Similarly, because this is a new area of research, we don't have any clear guidelines for avoiding gaming disorder, but given that heavy use seems to be a key risk factor for addiction, the recommendations already in place for putting reasonable limits on gaming time still hold—especially for individuals with autism.

What Do You Need to Know about Internet Access for Your Child with Autism?

Children with autism struggle to navigate the social world: they misread social cues, they misinterpret others' behavior, and they can get into relationships that aren't healthy or supportive. Because of this, it makes sense that a concern for many parents is unrestricted Internet access. According to national surveys by the Pew Foundation, as of 2018, 95% of American teens had a mobile phone or device (up from 73% in 2015), and 45% of teens report being on the Internet nearly constantly with another 44% reporting daily usage multiple times per day. By the time you read this, those numbers may be even higher. The main access point for many teens, their mobile phone, has many advantages for social connection. But for children inclined to avoid social contact, it may be isolating. Especially with handheld devices, it also privatizes the child's experience—making it difficult for parents to monitor what their children are doing online or via social media.

Mobile phone use interferes with attention and focus in the moment, simply by its distracting nature. We see this with adults who cannot focus during a meeting because they are distracted by an incoming text message. We see it in the scientific findings that a major cause of car accidents is drivers looking at their mobile device. We see it in college students distracted by their phone during a college lecture. We see it in pedestrians walking into traffic while staring at their phone. But as we noted earlier, long-term developmental effects on attentional control appear to be minor. The major concern that the clinical literature (and parents) report for children with autism is safety risks from the Internet itself: sexual victimization, cyberbullying, harassment or blackmail, and other more rare but worrying possibilities. Children who misjudge social context or social cues will be at heightened risk for stumbling into these scenarios or failing to manage the situation effectively if it occurs.

How frequently do these problems occur? No one is sure, but the best evidence is that serious problems, while common enough to warrant taking precautions, are far from universal—and tragic outcomes are reassuringly rare. This means you should be prudent but not alarmed. When they occur, the more serious risks of the Internet are related to excessive Internet or mobile usage. For example, two large recent studies reported that more mobile Internet use was associated with a greater chance of sexual or other victimization and riskier exposures (pornographic, violent, or extremist content). Other risk factors in the literature are lack of parental monitoring (child secrecy), children lacking awareness of risks, low child self-esteem, and a child's tendency to break rules.

Bottom line: While not all risky exposures are automatically harmful and the most tragic harms are rare, your child's mobile Internet use warrants your attention, and we recommend that you take the active precautions summarized below, particularly if you have a child who experiences the struggles with social interaction, social immaturity, and social naïveté that are common to autism.

✦

Action Steps to Reduce Internet Risks for Children with ASD

- Stay involved and communicate with your children about their online activity.
- Teach online safety: monitor your children's security settings and public disclosures.

- Make Internet access an activity that occurs in the family room or where you are present and not something that happens where you are unable to monitor.

- Separate out online gaming and recognize that it may have an important peer-connection aspect for some teens. If it does, then teach your child safety rules and make an agreement on reasonable amounts of use so it does not crowd out other important activities and social opportunities.

- Watch for signs of addiction (e.g., inability to handle limits on use, neglecting self-care or friends, neglecting homework, increased irritability)

TECHNOLOGY AND AUTISM INTERVENTIONS

A seemingly limitless number of technologically based interventions are touted for autism. Few are ready for prime time. Others won't necessarily address the core symptoms of autism but are accommodations that can be helpful for your child. For example, if your child has sound sensitivities, wearing headphones might make being in a range of environments more manageable or help him stay on task in a classroom setting. The technology for this can range from low tech (simple headphones) to high-tech noise-canceling devices. And there has been progress on making the degree to which the noise is canceled variable and controllable by the headphone wearer by setting (e.g., an airport) and type of auditory stimuli (e.g., child crying) variable by setting and type of auditory stimuli. These interventions can focus on addressing core challenges associated with autism, such as social skill acquisition through video modeling approaches.

As we discussed in Chapter 5, the empirical support for treatments of autism varies considerably. However, a meta-analysis of 18 randomized controlled studies evaluating the efficacy of different technology-based autism interventions for a variety of autism symptoms suggested that, collectively, the technological approaches resulted in greater gains than no-intervention control groups got. That's a low bar, but it suggests that there may be some promise in harnessing technology to intervene in autism.

This sort of makes sense, given that computer-based tasks can provide a degree of consistency helpful for an individual with autism. These tasks are free from social demands, which can be challenging, and they can build heavily on visual cues and can provide immediate, repeatable, and predictable responses—all things that research suggests are helpful for an individual with autism. So there is promise in these methods, with the caveat that computer-based tasks can isolate a child from the social world and we want to promote the opposite for your child with autism.

Here are the findings regarding some of the more common technology-based interventions that you are likely to encounter.

Alternative and Augmentative Communication Technology

Alternative and augmentative communication (AAC) is a broad category of interventions designed to assist with language and communication by supporting the transfer of visual or auditory cues. AAC has been investigated in autism since the 1980s, although technology has expanded the quality, reach, and price considerably over the years. Early low-tech AAC approaches included teaching individuals to use graphic boards—a person would point to a symbol on the board to communicate or hand over a graphic symbol in exchange for an activity or object. For example, if a child wanted a glass of milk, she would pull out her graphic board filled with images of objects and activities and simply point to the picture of the glass of milk. One of these low-tech approaches is called the Picture Exchange Communication System (PECS). Some research has shown it to be effective in supporting communication, but a recent randomized controlled trial indicated that children receiving PECS don't use verbal language more effectively following training. The important message here is that while PECS and AAC approaches can help children communicate, they don't appear to be effective at promoting spoken language.

High-tech versions of these approaches built on these concepts by actually generating speech sounds in response to the push of a button. In the 1990s and early 2000s, the technological devices that served this purpose were expensive and time-consuming to personalize, and carting around these devices could be stigmatizing too. Since then apps for handheld devices have made this technology relatively affordable, highly flexible, customizable, socially acceptable, and easy to transport. And they still promote communication for requesting needs and wants—but they still do not promote the verbal use of language. Nor do they address any of the core challenges of autism such as difficulties in social interaction or restricted behaviors.

> Research has shown that AAC can help your child communicate wants and needs in the moment but not that it will promote the child's use of spoken language afterward.

If you decide to investigate AAC to promote your child's communication, be sure it's the right kind, which can only be determined through a careful, methodological, clinical process with a provider who has expertise in autism, communication, and AAC interventions. This provider can ensure an appropriate fit for your child's needs and the appropriate features of the AAC approach and provide clear instruction on how to effectively incorporate it into the existing treatment program. Even though these apps can be downloaded in under a minute to your own device whenever you want, the use of an AAC app should not replace appropriate clinical care promoting communication.

Technology-Based Programs for Academic Instruction

Using technology to teach academic skills to children with autism is not a new idea. Unfortunately, it's also not a very well-studied idea. An early study published in 1973 reported the results from using a series of computer-based games to link letters to speech sounds. In one of the simple computer games, a child pressed a letter, and the computer would say it and show a picture of an object spelled with that as its first letter. Few conclusions could be drawn from that study given its methodological limitations, and since then not many well-designed studies have researched such technology-based interventions A recent review of all such studies published since the mid-1990s identified only three quality studies. The takeaway is that teachers should be cautious when using technology-based interventions to teach academic skills for children with ASD. We just don't really know if they're more or less effective than traditional approaches.

Technology-Based Approaches to Teaching Emotion Recognition

Technology-based approaches to teaching emotion recognition skills to people with autism have a little bit more scientific support than interventions for academic instruction, although the literature is still relatively new. The rationale behind applying technology specifically to teaching emotion recognition is that with technology a practitioner can control distractions that occur naturally in our social environment by either freezing or covering parts of the environment. That way, a practitioner can help focus the learner's attention on areas of interest such as the eyes or mouth, which are the parts of the face where we can learn to recognize emotions. Then the practitioner can coach the learner on what to attend to and how to make sense of the available information.

A large number of studies have examined this topic. A recent systematic review identified 285 studies published since 2000 focused on technology-based interventions specifically examining emotion recognition in ASD. After identifying studies that don't directly investigate the effectiveness of technological interventions and those trials hampered by methodological limitations, the authors of this review winnowed the list down to 15 studies, including 382 participants, to include in their review. Ten of those were clinical trials, and the remainder were single-subject designs (studies where only one participant is included). The scientists concluded there is preliminary evidence that technology-based interventions focused on learning facial features with specific coaching instruction can improve emotion recognition. However, the studies that were reviewed included wide age ranges, small samples, widely differing technologies, distinct emotion recognition training protocols, and different measurements of effectiveness. As a result, while the evidence suggests that the technology can be effective, we should be cautious in how we use these technologies.

> There is preliminary evidence that technology can help teach children emotion recognition skills, but we need to be cautious in applying it until it's studied further.

Video Modeling and Video Self-Modeling Interventions

Fifty years ago, pioneering psychologist Albert Bandura showed that children learn a range of skills simply by observing others, rather than through personal experience. Importantly, he found that children will imitate others' behavior even without rewards, will do so in settings other than those where they first saw the behavior, and will usually imitate those they view as competent and similar to themselves in some way, such as age, physical appearance, ethnicity, and so forth.

Video modeling uses Bandura's discoveries in interventions for autism. Typically, a child watches a demonstration of a targeted behavior and then imitates that behavior. In video self-modeling the learner watches a video of herself successfully performing the behavior. Video self-modeling takes particular advantage of Bandura's findings in that the model can't get any more similar to the learner and the learner gets to see herself successfully performing the behavior so she knows that she can do it. It promotes greater likelihood that she'll imitate the behavior.

As one might imagine, it is pretty easy to generate videos demonstrating behaviors you want your child to learn. The video app on your phone lets you do that in almost any situation. But it's more difficult to generate a video of your child successfully completing a behavior that you want her to learn. Fortunately research has shown that both types of video modeling not only promote skills but also that the skills acquired are maintained over time and generalized to multiple settings. The skills that have been examined have included social communication skills, such as initiating and responding to social interactions and taking others' perspectives; functional skills, such as meal preparation, doing the laundry, cooking, and self-care; and behavioral skills, such as play. A meta-analytic study of video modeling including 42 studies and 126 individuals with autism found that while video modeling was most effective for elementary-school-age children, it was effective across all age groups and was equally effective for boys and girls.

Virtual Reality

As you may know, considering how rapidly virtual reality tools are emerging, virtual reality is an artificial environment created by a computer through exposure to stimuli (such as sights and sounds) that allows you to interact with and partially determine what happens in that environment. Augmented virtual reality is a type of virtual reality in which additional information is laid over the actual environment and experienced through headsets or a smartphone or even, now, through glasses. Virtual reality has already been used to enhance health care generally and mental health in particular, including the treatment of phobias, posttraumatic stress disorder, and compulsive behaviors. As you might imagine, there has been interest in exploring virtual reality to treat autism as well.

One of the primary strengths of virtual reality is that it allows for the careful construction of real-life scenarios that provide a perfect place to practice either social or language skills in a safe, therapist-controlled environment. Additionally, data can be collected in this environment, allowing a therapist to quantify progress or skills development to inform the therapeutic regimen. Additionally, incentives specific to a child's interests can be incorporated in the treatment, or the experience can have a gaming-type quality to it, encouraging practicing of targeted skills that can be rewarded in the same way playing Fortnite or Minecraft can be rewarding. The ease of application offered by the increasingly available augmented-reality glasses makes it more and more likely that we'll be able to incorporate these supports into everyday life.

A recent systematic review of virtual reality interventions in autism, published in 2018, suggested virtual reality approaches have promise, but the evidence is still limited. The review included 650 participants across 31 studies addressing treatment to improve attention, social skills, emotion recognition, daily living skills, communication, physical activity, and fears. The scientists found moderate evidence for its effectiveness at improving skills across those domains. Improvements have been reported in social skills and emotion recognition skills, but the methodologies and approaches in the empirical studies vary considerably, making it difficult to draw strong conclusions. The takeaway message is that you are likely to see a massive increase in the number of applications and studies of virtual reality for the treatment of autism, and widespread use of virtual reality interventions, but for now, you are best advised to save your money until these new tools are better tested.

Social Robotics

Robotics, and specifically socially assistive robotics, provide aid through social interaction, as opposed to physical interaction. In areas of rehabilitation medicine, socially assistive robotics have helped out with tasks such as encouraging patients to stick to a therapy program through verbal encouragement or reminders for appointments, to take medicine, or to complete daily living tasks for patients with dementia. In nursing homes, socially assistive robots have been used in the common areas to promote social interaction among residents. In autism, robotics have been used as an intervention tool to improve eye contact, imitation skills, emotion recognition ability, joint attention skills, and turn-taking and social interactions.

It's possible that social robots are effective in autism because they simplify the input people receive in human interactions, making it easier to process information, interpret social cues, and develop social skills. We don't have many quality studies yet, but one recent systematic review concluded that participants with autism tended to perform better on measures of eye contact, sharing attention, imitation, and verbal responding and showed fewer repetitive behaviors when interacting with a robot compared to a person. Although this is not the case for all studies with robots, the scientists concluded that when interacting with socially assistive robotics, individuals with autism showed more prosocial behaviors, suggesting that robotics can help therapists engage with individuals with autism, so this technology might support therapies. The takeaway is that robotics are not a replacement for a therapist, but a tool that therapists may use to augment therapies that we know are effective, such as behaviorally based interventions.

◈

Take-Home Points

- New high-tech methods of treating autism are fascinating—and in some cases quite promising—but most are not yet ready for prime time. Keep an eye on these, but don't spend money on them yet. The next few years are likely to see numerous new developments.

- Computer and mobile screens and the Internet are here to stay, and it's important to stay tuned in to your child's media and Internet use. Technological devices provide today's young people with social connection and unlimited information, but they also introduce unique risks for children with autism, particularly with regard to opening the door to victimization and restricting opportunities for direct social interaction. While the harmful effect of screen media on the development of attention appears to be slight, other risks are real and warrant following the steps outlined in this chapter to keep your child with autism safe from the secondary harms that can occur.

9

ADOLESCENCE AND AUTISM

One of the things that we all know about children is that they don't stay children forever. They quickly turn into teenagers, and then they grow up to be adults. At each stage along the way there are new challenges (and new joys), and that's exactly the same for your child with autism. There will be ups and downs as the social world becomes more and more complex through adolescence and as the demands of the social world change again during and following the transition into adulthood.

During the teenage years, your child will be navigating a social world with rapidly changing social norms, which will likely differ from those at home and from what was expected of your son or daughter in elementary school. Your teen will face increased demands on her ability to manage her time and organize her materials and schedule. And your child will face new complications around sexuality and romantic relationships.

Imagine Jonah, a child one of us worked with. In the cafeteria line, he would bite his lips and crack his knuckles while he waited to order his lunch. The other children milling around him would joke and chide one another, eagerly waiting for a needed respite from academic concentration. Jonah instead would watch the cafeteria lady closely, searching for a clue that would help him decipher this mayhem. Later he would tell me that he employed Jedi mind tricks to make his fellow students move more slowly, hoping to delay the moment when he would have to choose where to sit: "This is not the carton of milk you are looking for; choose a different one." His efforts were always futile; he would advance efficiently through the line and have no choice but to cross the threshold into the lunchroom. He would survey the room. Again, he shared that he would hope for miracles—maybe one of his friends from chess club would have been switched into his lunch period. After failing to find one of his few friends, he started to scan the room again. This second time he would be searching for the oasis of an unoccupied table. He explained that the days at empty tables were easier; he could eat quickly and retreat to the library or computer lab. On most days he wasn't so fortunate and had to join classmates at one of the partially filled tables. Fortunately, he wasn't teased much. Rather, his approach often went unnoticed. Maybe one of his classmates would greet him or offer a token "What's up?" More often, they just gave him a glance and a smile and then continued with their conversation. Jonah would smile back, perhaps fumble over a reply, and then quietly eat his lunch. Sometimes peers tried to engage him in conversation about the latest cool clothes or what someone was discussing on social media the night before, but the discussion always seemed to fizzle despite Jonah's best efforts. Jonah couldn't come up with what to say quickly enough; sometimes he took mental notes on the conversations going on around him. He was always mystified by the fluidity of the other children's statements, their quick gestures, and their expressive faces. It was as if they knew a language he had never learned. He found sitting at a lunch table profoundly anxiety provoking (what if he mangled yet *another* conversation?) and, after the fact, felt sad.

Jonah's attention to the social world, despite his limited ability to rapidly and fluidly navigate it, proved to be helpful for him. Additionally, his mother's checking in with him after school and his strong relationship with a therapist helped him organize his reflections on his day and at times practice the skills he needed in a safe environment, so that he could more successfully navigate his way through high school. And indeed, he did. Jonah ended up graduating with his classmates and attended an area community college where he could excel academically and continue to get the support he needed from his parents to tackle the day-to-day complex interactions.

Let's add to the typical high school day of navigating not only the lunchroom but also the locker room and many hallway social interactions the need to navigate many class and other transitions, which we know are challenging for teens with autism. For some teens, classes are held in different rooms, teachers rotate, and the schedule—and the expectations—vary from day to day. Not only does that mean regulating the emotional challenges of not having a set routine and of the multiple transitions, but it also means meeting the cognitive challenge: having to remember where to be and when, having to move quickly from topic to topic, and needing to have all the appropriate materials ready. It's not easy. The typical high school weekday is effectively an executive functioning iron man triathlon for kids with ASD.

Across all of this is layered the development of sexuality. Your teenager's body is changing and maturing even though social development and behavior may not be developing at the same pace. Making sense of those maturational changes exceeds the typical teenager's grasp to begin with; it is even more difficult for your child with atypical emotional, social, and behavioral challenges. And navigating that sexual development within the context of rapidly changing social norms and subtle signals can feel insurmountable to the teen (and perhaps to you).

But it is surmountable. Just like a preschool or elementary school child with autism, your teen will have joys and fun times interspersed with these harder moments and challenges. With the tried-and-true tips, techniques, and suggestions embedded in this chapter, based on findings we've extracted from the currently exploding scientific literature on this topic and guided by our years of working with families, we hope you will have more tools to navigate this period.

And then your teenager will become an adult. Obviously this change will not take place overnight but is a gradual transition. Increasingly, we recognize that in our society, the "transition ages" from about 18 to 25 are a critical developmental period. This may be especially true for young people with ASD. Thus, early adulthood brings yet another stage of joys and challenges. Marie, a parent in this situation, told one of us that when her son Roger turned 21 and was no longer able to be in the public school system they felt like they "fell off a cliff."

Why did she say that? Marie was faced with a new medical and psychological service system for Roger, who had both autism and intellectual disability. Once he finished high school, these services were fewer, more dispersed, and more difficult to navigate. She had to scour the community for meaningful, inclusive activities for her son now that school was no longer an option for how he would spend his days. She needed to familiarize herself with the legal and financial systems so she could ensure that her son would be supported through adulthood and, as she shared tearfully, after she was no longer available to take care of him.

Yet for those who make the transition to an appropriate life situation, early adulthood can be a positive period. While the scientific literature suggests that for the majority of individuals with autism young adulthood is incredibly challenging, with significant hardships in employment, housing, and mental health concerns, this is not the case for all individuals. For a solid minority, early adulthood is a time to pursue one's own interests, succeed in secondary education, or enjoy family relationships without the stress of the complex adolescent social world.

Sally, whose daughter Anna had autism and intellectual disability, had that experience. Anna was able to move into housing in the community supported by state funding. Sally felt that for the first time in 21 years she was able to sleep the whole night through. But this didn't help just her. Anna also seemed to benefit from the new setting, independence, stimulation, and community. Their relationship improved too. Sally used her newfound energy to connect with her daughter doing activities together during the day that she had never had energy for in the past. Of course, that type of placement isn't always available or workable. Other parents find that the transition period into early adulthood is no harder or easier than any other period, just different. For Arthur, graduation from high school meant enrolling in a community college and living in his parents' basement. His father, Daryl, supported Arthur in much the same way he did during high school: helping organize his days, homework, and activities; helping ensure he got on the public bus so that he'd make his way to campus each day; and serving as the "quarterback" for his son's services—social skills group, vocational training, and individual therapy for anxiety.

Although all three families had to learn new systems and address new challenges, they also shared some of the same celebrations: their young adult's successful participation in a community rumba dance class, joy at sitting in the passenger seat on a cross-country drive, or high school graduation.

There have been ups and downs for all the parents we've worked with, and for their maturing child, when that youth has transitioned into adulthood. Adolescence hands youth with ASD two developmental tasks:

navigating the teen years and preparing for the transition to early adulthood. We'll walk you through the preparatory steps in the remainder of this chapter; in Chapter 10, we'll focus on navigating the early adult period itself. The teenage years confront the youth with fast-changing social norms and "coolness," new demands on time management and organizational skills, and profound developmental changes related to social and physical aspects of sexuality and romantic relationships. Fortunately, you have a number of resources you can use, starting during the teen years, that will help you and your teen manage the downs so that there are more ups than downs during those transition years into early adulthood.

FIRST RESOURCE: DEVELOPMENT OF ADAPTIVE SKILLS

A number of longitudinal studies have now shown that one of the key predictors of success in adulthood for those on the autism spectrum is developing what are called "adaptive skills." Adaptive skills, also called daily living skills, are the skills you need to be able to live independently and take care of yourself. These include skills such as learning to cook a meal, manage a budget, dress appropriately, use proper hygiene, clean your room, use transportation, and show up for work or school on time. These "life skills" take time to learn, and too often academics take priority over these types of skills. Thus, it is essential that you as a parent help your adolescent learn these skills by focusing on them at home, in school, and in the community.

> Take every opportunity to teach your child adaptive skills or "daily living skills" during adolescence—it will pay off in the transition to adulthood.

Fortunately, you don't need an advanced degree to help a child or adolescent learn daily living skills. You can start early by expecting your child or adolescent to use manners, take the dishes from the table, help clean and put dishes away, help with laundry, and so on. These types of chores will help build a foundation for independent living, whether in a dorm, group home, or apartment. Similarly, you can teach your adolescent how to prepare and eat healthy foods, brush his teeth, take a regular shower, and choose the appropriate clothing for the weather and activities of the day. Your adolescent will especially appreciate learning how to function independently in the community, such as ordering food at a restaurant, checking the time, saving money and making purchases, and learning to ride the bus.

Typical kids often learn these skills by watching and imitating others. However, one of the difficulties kids with ASD have is "imitating" others. First, your child might not be paying attention to others due to a lack of interest. Second, she might miss some of the nuances that make the difference between executing a skill well and missing it. For example, she might know how to buy a bus ticket but not know that she has to be paying attention so she doesn't miss her stop. The point is that each of these skills likely will need to be taught explicitly and practiced. It's a good idea to begin working on them as early as possible, even in early childhood. That way, by the time your adolescent is thinking about what she plans to do after high school, she will be better prepared for that next stage of life.

Your teen might not be naturally motivated to learn adaptive skills. It's OK to set up a reward system for doing chores and using good hygiene. If your adolescent has an IEP, it's a good idea to incorporate daily living skills into his IEP goals. This could include learning how to ask for help, monitor time throughout the day, choose a healthy lunch, and so on. Adaptive skills are part of everyday life and occur in all settings throughout the day. Use every opportunity to teach these skills to your adolescent to help prepare him for the next stage of life.

SECOND RESOURCE: EDUCATION IN SOCIAL SKILLS

The key here is explicit teaching of what seems to us to be intuitive. While neurotypical children develop social skills fluidly and without conscious direction (we call that "implicit" learning), the individual with ASD learns "explicitly"—through verbalizing. Thankfully, that can work!

We've learned through much research and trial and error that we can teach and promote social skills and social behavior. Some children will be able to learn those social skills successfully through methods discussed in Chapter 5, such as therapies based on applied behavior analysis

(ABA). By reinforcing your young child's attention to the social world, those methods help the child or teen attend more regularly and soak in that valuable social information that helps him learn about emotions and communication—key parts of the social world. As we noted, by scaffolding your child's social interaction, ABA-based therapies teach him to navigate social interactions successfully. Over time and repeated successful practice, your child will develop the skills to both use social skills and track social cues so that his learning of social norms and communications becomes a lifelong process.

But for most of you, there is still more work for your youngster to do during the teen years. Maybe the availability of ABA for your child was limited when she was younger. The good news is that it's not too late for your teen to benefit—we can still apply those principles of rewarding social behavior, but now we combine that with even more explicit explaining and teaching of social cues and norms through particular social skills curricula. (Validated and specific manualized programs are available in major university-based centers and autism clinics; see the Resources for a list of such clinics.) If they are not available in your area, you may still find a counselor who provides the same method and can help you transfer it to home.

These social skills programs range greatly in their scope and delivery method, but they typically involve a didactic (classroom-like teaching/ explaining) component regarding what the value and purpose of a particular social skill component is, the opportunity to practice that skill in structured and unstructured ways, and explicit reinforcement and recognition for successful use of that skill.

For example, one session of a group-based social skills program may include a brief outline of the value of back-and-forth conversation and what that looks like. There may then be an activity such as conversation pong, where partners have to practice having a conversation about a particular topic while passing a ping pong ball between them. The receiver of the ping pong ball can't throw it back until he makes a statement that builds on the thrower's comment. During that activity, the clinician would reinforce success in learning the skill through an explicit point system and verbal recognition of the natural contingencies (e.g., "Joseph, you get a point for asking what kind of pizza Billy liked when he said he liked pizza . . . and did you see how excited Jarod got when he was able to tell you about mushroom pizza?") Then, following the activity, during an unstructured portion of the session, such as during a snack, the clinician reinforces successful use of that social skill during naturalistic interactions.

Those are the elements typical of social skills curricula, but these programs can vary in setting (in the clinic or at school), in frequency (once a week or several times a week), size (dyad or group), scope (focus on broad skills or just one aspect such as theory of mind), who is involved (child-only group or child and caregiver concurrent groups), and who is the active agent (clinician delivered or peer mediated).

A recent summary of data from 19 randomized controlled trials of clinician-facilitated, group-based social skills interventions for teens with autism reveals a modest effect of these types of social skills interventions on social competence. Interestingly, the degree of effectiveness of social skills interventions for people with autism is similar to the effectiveness of social skills training for individuals with ADHD and schizophrenia, but much larger than the effect size for schoolwide or afterschool programs for the general school population. This suggests that the efficacy of this type of intervention is really specific to those with particular challenges in developing specific skills involved in navigating the social world.

However, the greatest impact of social skills training was on the participants' knowledge of social skills—the participants tended to learn social skills and reported that they had learned them, but not necessarily that they used these new skills. This may be why parents and teachers who evaluated the effects didn't report observing much increase in social skill competence.

> *Ongoing social skills training is invaluable to teens facing new social challenges now and into adulthood.*

Besides clinician-facilitated training, there are interventions supported through the inclusion of typical peer models. The rationale behind these approaches is that by having typically developing peers model or prompt particular social skills, such as in a school setting, the participants with autism can learn the skills in an inclusive environment, and the interaction can promote further social engagement between students with autism and their peers. Recently a review of 14 studies suggested that this is a promising approach for promoting improved social inter-actions between students with ASD and their peers in school settings. But it's important to note that each study included only one teen with ASD. Still, the skills taught were being used in the schools outside of that social skills class setting and were maintained over time. While this peer-based approach to social skills instruction is still relatively new, it appears to show promise.

THIRD RESOURCE:
TIME MANAGEMENT AND ORGANIZATIONAL SKILLS

Transitioning between classes, staying on top of homework, and navigat-ing the halls, lockers, and schedule changes are all part of daily life in high school. This challenge has two components. The first concerns the practical demands of time and organization, which rely heavily on execu-tive functioning abilities. These are abilities that, as we discussed earlier in Chapter 4, science tells us are often developing differently and are less efficient in this situation for children with autism.

The second challenge concerns difficulties with changes, transitions, and disruptions to routine. This, as we discussed when talking about the concept of insistence on sameness in Chapter 2, is part and parcel of autism. These difficulties can result in emotions that might be difficult to manage in the moment and challenging behaviors that result from that emotional dysregulation. We'll discuss action items to tackle that in the next section on emotion regula-tion.

High school presents a host of new time management and task-juggling challenges to all teens. For those with ASD, it's even more important to learn organizational and planning skills and use them every day.

Addressing homework, schedule changes, and multiple class assign-ments requires time management and executive functioning skills— abilities such as planning and hold-ing different ideas in your mind so you can think about them. Executive functioning skills are critical for managing time, learning, and doing things like homework. A number of books help promote time manage-ment for students, so we won't spend too much time delving into this, but in the box on the facing page we highlight some of the key executive functioning tools that you (and most important, your teenager) can use for a successful learning experience in high school.

FOURTH RESOURCE: EMOTION REGULATION STRATEGIES

Teens face a lot of situations that provoke emotional reactions that exceed their ability to manage. As we mentioned above, daily high school life requires transitions and regular disruptions to routines; sensory stimuli, such as loud noises or flickering fluorescent lights, can be overwhelming; and the rapidly changing social world can be nearly impossible to follow. All of these typical adolescent situations can tax a teen's ability to regulate his emotional experience. For these challenges, however, there are some straightforward actionable approaches you can take.

Emotional Challenges Associated with Transitions

Dealing with unexpected changes or disruptions to routines and transitioning from one activity to another (even as part of one's daily routine) can be difficult for many teens with autism. For some, disruptions to routine or rapid transitions between classes can result in anxiety or oppositional behavior or even a tantrum. These emotional experiences can be very difficult to manage or resolve in the moment. It's best to prevent the emotional meltdown before it begins. Helping your child anticipate and plan for unexpected changes can help your teenager navigate transitions. Doing that means paying more attention to what is happening at your child's school than you might have planned on for your high school student, so that you know when assemblies are occurring or when the math teacher will be absent. The easiest way to know what is going on for your high schooler is to establish a good relationship with your student's special education teacher, school psychologist, or, if your child is not receiving any additional supports through your school, with a homeroom teacher or other engaged teacher on your child's schedule. Nowadays, with e-mail and school websites, it's easier to connect and find out what is happening with your child's schedule.

To facilitate the need for rapid transitions between one class and

Successful Time Management Tips
for High School Students with Autism

1. Make a to-do list every day. Start at the top of the list with the most important things and do those first. Check off the tasks as you complete them.

2. Follow the Premack principle, which states that more probable behaviors will reinforce less probable behaviors. This means when there are things to be done, start with the tasks that are the least desirable and work your way up. Simply put, if your child likes playing video games, make sure that happens after he completes his chores. Even when both things aren't particularly fun, ordering them with the least desirable task, or the one least likely to get done, first will increase the likelihood that both will be done. If your child prefers math over reading even a little bit, having her complete her reading homework first will increase the likelihood that she'll finish both.

3. Use an agenda. Have a master schedule that not only includes homework but also has other activities penciled in, including fun time and leisure activities.

4. Have your child use spare minutes wisely. If there is homework to be done and there is some free time while waiting for the school bus, that's the perfect time to do it.

5. Figure out when your child works his best. If his brain can handle math in the morning, he'll be more efficient doing math homework in the morning than at the end of the day.

6. Start assignments early. Getting started on an assignment always works better than waiting until the last minute.

7. Break tasks into manageable chunks. For many children with autism, a large assignment can seem overwhelming, but if you help them break down the assignment into manageable chunks, they can systematically chip away at each piece.

8. Have your child spend a few minutes reviewing her notes every day. Easier said than done, but reviewing notes at the end of each day means less actual time studying come exam time.

9. Make sure your child gets a good night's sleep. We spent nearly a

(continued)

whole chapter espousing the virtues of sleep, so we won't linger on this one, but suffice it to say that with better sleep comes more efficiency.

10. Establish good homework hygiene. That means having a setting free of distractions, establishing a homework routine and schedule, and taking care to stick to that so there aren't incoming phone calls or text messages or siblings interrupting that time.

11. Work in shorter bursts. Our brains get tired and we don't concentrate as well after 30–45 minutes of work. Plan for a short break to get up, walk around, move the body for a few minutes to refresh, and then begin working again. These breaks will actually make your child more efficient.

another, your teen can use a straightforward approach that includes the same types of things that helped her when she was younger. Having a written or visual schedule can help an individual anticipate what is happening during any given day. Color coding can help highlight changes in the schedule.

Labeling the schedule by incorporating your child's interests can be helpful. For example, 16-year-old Allen liked Marvel comics, so he labeled each day of his school week schedule with a different superhero. It was a simple task to paste a picture of his superhero at the top of his printed class schedule, and it promoted his interest in looking at and using his schedule. It also allowed parents, teachers, or counselors to scaffold his anticipatory coping: they could ask him what Iron Man would do on Thursdays when math class came after physical education instead of lunch like it did every other day of the week; how would Iron Man deal with that change to his routine? Allen could use this method to visualize and anticipate and cope.

Other supports could include working with the school through an IEP or 504 plan. One tactic here is to add to the plan to allow for transitioning time to the next class before or after the actual class transition time. This will allow your child to move through the halls in a less sensory stimulating environment. Or your child may benefit from a visual timer on her desk to help her track the time to transition to the next activity. School personnel will likely have other potential supports like this that they can offer once the goal is named.

Emotional Challenges Associated with Sensory Overstimulation

As we've discussed throughout this book, sensory sensitivities are part of the diagnosis of autism. These sensitivities vary by child, but often we see sensitivities to loud sounds (e.g., fire alarms), particular sounds (e.g., buzzing fans), touch (e.g., unexpected bump by another student in a crowded hallway), sights (e.g., fluorescent lights), and smells (e.g., particular foods). These sensory sensitivities can be distracting, be stressful, and cause emotional outbursts. Accommodations for these types of sensory sensitivities can be a practical intervention to reduce emotional dysregulation for your child. Accommodations can include using earplugs or headphones, using sunglasses or simply wearing a hat to block out brighter lights, and having a quiet room available to take a break from the sensory stimulation. By working with your child's school you can incorporate accommodations like these, ones that are specific to your child's challenges, directly into her individualized education plan.

Emotional Challenges More Broadly

There are a couple of therapeutic approaches you can take to managing emotions. First, there is considerable evidence in the literature supporting the effectiveness of CBT in managing anxiety and depression. Applying CBT to multiple emotional problems also has support from randomized controlled trials. When applied to autism, there is similar support for its effectiveness. It's important to note that CBT-based therapies require sufficient cognitive abilities to reflect on one's thoughts and behaviors and motivation to change. Many psychologists use CBT to teach children, adolescents, and adults to learn to manage their emotions. This includes helping adolescents who have emotional outbursts or whose emotional response seems out of proportion to the situation, as well as those who are struggling with anxiety and depression. If this is an area of concern for you, consider contacting a psychologist who works with adolescents with ASD in your area.

The second approach that is starting to receive some support in the literature is teaching mindfulness. In mindfulness-based therapies, the focus is on training a person to focus his attention on the present moment in a nonjudgmental way ("I recognize that I'm feeling angry, but that feeling is neither good nor bad. It just is the feeling that I'm having"). That focus may be on sensations in the body, thoughts, or feelings, but regardless of the focus, the sensations or cognitions are not to influence behavior in that moment. The active ingredient of mindfulness-based therapies involves increased emotional awareness and the associated improved emotional regulation. A 2018 review highlights mindfulness as an alternative for teens and adults with autism because during high-stress situations the skills taught by CBT therapies can be hard to implement in the moment. Although there is still limited empirical support for mindfulness-based therapies, this approach shows promise.

Mindfulness offers a relatively new way for teens on the spectrum to manage emotions in the moment.

FIFTH RESOURCE:
SUPPORTING SEXUALITY IN YOUR TEENAGER WITH AUTISM

Early claims that individuals with autism were asexual were a myth: it is well established that most individuals with autism very clearly want romantic and sexual relationships despite outward behavior that may not convey that. Just like their typically developing peers, adolescents (and adults) with autism show the whole range of typical to problematic social behaviors.

However, there are some critical differences for teens with ASD. Teens with autism tend to have greater difficulties adapting to the physical changes associated with puberty and tend to experience more anxiety, distress, and loneliness than their typical peers; this transition is particularly problematic for girls with ASD.

The research also tells us that your child's sexual development is likely to be different from that of his peers. Reasons for that include the social challenges that are part and parcel of autism, reduced opportunities for formal sex education, and an increased rate of diversity in sexual orientation and sexual identity satisfaction among today's youth. Most important, although your child with ASD will experience key differences and challenges unique to him, avenues and supports can be put in place to increase the likelihood of a healthy sexual development and identity.

The first reason that your child's sexual development will differ from that of her peers is tied specifically to the social communication and interaction challenges, which can affect her ability to use social information and thus to keep and maintain friendships. Fewer peer relationships and less relationship experience mean fewer opportunities to practice and learn how to use social information to guide behavior—a kind of self-reinforcing circle.

The same logic holds in the challenge of navigating the development of sexuality and sexual behaviors—difficulty tracking the social cues and fewer opportunities to practice those skills, in a self-reinforcing loop. This is reflected in what the research says about rates of sexually problematic behavior in ASD. Systematic reviews report higher rates of problematic behaviors for individuals with autism, such as public masturbation, indecent exposure, voyeurism, and fetishism. These are likely related to failure to notice social norms and expectations. Now, most youth with ASD still don't engage in these behaviors. By "higher rates" we mean compared to what is observed in the typical population. For example, surveys of young adults with autism and intellectual disability suggest that 25–30% engaged in inappropriate sexual behaviors at least once. Engaging in behaviors that fall out of the social norm makes sense if you're not able to use clues in your social environment to help guide your own behavior. If you're not able to pick up those clues through observation, it's critical to get that information in other, more formal ways. However, unfortunately, formal educational approaches are happening less for students with autism rather than more. Fortunately, there are ways to fill that gap:

Communication

First and foremost is establishing and maintaining open communication with your teen. Talking about sex is not easy for many people, but doing so in an open, calm manner is critical for keeping communication lines clear. Having clear lines of communication with your teenager means that you can be available to answer questions and provide education, feedback, and guidance, just as you would with any topic facing a teenager, from driving to studying. That open communication will mean that you can help promote healthy sexual behavior and positive behavior in romantic relationships and answer questions about gender identity. As difficult as it may be, it is triply critical for your child because your child is not able to pick up information about sexuality and romantic behavior informally or formally elsewhere. Essentially it is either you or the Internet. And, we're going to put our money on you. If you're not comfortable with these types of conversations, then seek out those who are, such as a clinician with expertise in autism and adolescence.

Among the topics that you or another trusted adult will want to discuss with your adolescent are (1) understanding the difference between public and private behavior (including the topic of masturbation); (2) who should be able to touch your child and where; (3) proper and improper names of body parts and when it is appropriate to use these terms; (4) the concept of personal space; (5) how to avoid situations that are high risk for sexual or physical abuse, and what to do if someone does something inappropriate or harmful; and (6) what dating is and how to do it. These are not one-time conversations but rather an ongoing, open dialogue with some topics visited frequently. Hopefully, your adolescent's school will offer educational programs about sexuality, as discussed next.

Sex Ed

The research shows, unfortunately, that your child with autism is less likely to get the same degree and type of sexual health education as other teens. The reason for this discrepancy is unclear. It has been hypothesized that problematic behaviors and attentional problems in the school limit opportunities in the classroom, and so sexual education is dropped from the schedule in favor of other parts of the curriculum. Another proposed reason is that teachers are not comfortable providing sexual health information for students with autism. Turns out that surveys indicate this is true for parents as well—so you're not alone if you are wondering how to go about having conversations on sexuality with your teen with ASD.

So, where are teens with autism getting their information about sexuality? Research indicates that teens and young adults with autism are looking to the Internet for sexual education to fill the gap. While some of that information could be appropriate, accurate, and constructive, it's just as likely, perhaps more likely, that it's inaccurate and problematic. So having fewer opportunities for informal (e.g., through observing social behavior) and formal (e.g., sexual education at school) sexual health education puts your child doubly at a disadvantage relative to typically developing peers.

> *Open, direct communication about sexuality and autism-specific sex education programs are essential to your teen.*

The good news is that in response to the observed lack of sexual health education teens with autism are receiving, autism-specific programs are beginning to be developed. One such program is called Tackling Teenage Training. There is no empirical evidence to support one program over the other, but participating in a program that provides clear, accurate information and promotes communication may prove particularly helpful. Given the higher rates of sexual orientation diversity and gender dysphoria that researchers have found in individuals with autism, such a program could be incredibly important for your child, especially if it helps promote a healthy sexual identity that best fits with your child's self-concept and not one that is shaped simply by perceptions of what is socially acceptable in the general population. (Gender dysphoria refers to distress resulting from a disconnect between one's assigned gender and one's own experienced gender coupled with the persistent desire to be of another gender.)

Take Questions about Sexual Identity Seriously

Much of the research on sexual orientation and gender dysphoria in people with ASD has focused on teens and young adults with autism who have cognitive abilities falling in or above the average range and who were able to communicate their sexual orientation and experience of their gender identity, so it's important to consider these findings in that context. We have less insight into the experience of individuals with autism and intellectual disability who are less able to articulate their inner experience.

A recent systematic review and meta-analysis of studies involving anonymous surveys of over 1,000 young adults with autism found higher rates of homosexuality and bisexuality than in the neurotypical population. Study rates vary, but between 15 and 35% of participants with autism reported having an exclusive homosexual or bisexual orientation. This is significantly higher than the reported rates in the neurotypical population in the United States and Britain, which at the time of those studies in the early 2000s were 4.6% and 5.4%, respectively.

Although there are fewer studies that examine sexual orientation across genders, the existing studies suggest that this pattern is more pronounced for females than males. Why is this? Some theories suggest that because of limited opportunities and experience with romantic partners, individuals with autism may not identify gender as a relevant characteristic for choosing a partner, may have a limited understanding of what the concept of sexual orientation means, or might not understand or care about what sexual orientation norms exist in society. Given recent advances in the neurobiology of autism, such as what we discussed in Chapter 4, some scientists hypothesize reduced rates of heterosexuality in females with autism might result from elevated rates of testosterone during fetal development; however, this hypothesis does not account for higher rates of homosexuality in males with autism.

> Issues of gender identity and sexual orientation come up more often for teens with ASD than others and should be sensitively addressed.

As we mentioned above, gender dysphoria refers to distress associated with a discrepancy between one's assigned gender and one's own experienced gender along with the persistent desire to be of another gender. Although research into gender dysphoria is relatively new, science tells us that individuals with autism have a much higher rate of gender dysphoria than the typical population. In the typical population the rate of gender dysphoria is somewhere between 1 in 10,000 and 1 in 20,000 birth-assigned males and 1 in 30,000 to 50,000 females. Like the diagnostic rates of autism, the rates of gender dysphoria are on the rise. It is unclear if this rise reflects a true increase or simply reflects that transgender care and support is more culturally accepted and visible. The rate of gender dysphoria in autism varies by study, but a recent systematic review of studies of autism and gender dysphoria including almost 1,500 children and adolescents suggests co-occurrence rates between 3 and 14%. This is remarkably higher than the typical population rate. This area of research is very new, and there is no agreement on why there is an overrepresentation of gender dysphoria in autism. Several proposals are out there, but none are definite. One idea is that it relates to increased exposure to androgens in utero, a reflection of rigid thinking patterns or preoccupations, or the result of a differential gender identity developmental pattern. However, these are all speculative; none of these proposed hypotheses have any specific evidence to support them. Further, there is little scientific consensus on the diagnosis and support for gender dysphoria and autism. More research clearly needs to be done in this area so that we can develop tools to provide the most appropriate support for this unique population.

For now, you will need to check your own assumptions about your child's sexual orientation as there is a greater likelihood that your child might have questions about this, and you'll want to support her. Relatedly, while the majority of children with autism do not struggle with distress associated with their assigned gender, many do. Do not hesitate to seek help from a clinician with expertise in autism. The diagnostic process regarding gender dysphoria is complicated in autism, and supports and options for individuals should be reviewed with a clinician who has expertise in autism and an understanding of the specific needs of this unique group of individuals. For a summary of action steps you can take, see the box on the following page.

SIXTH RESOURCE: THE TRANSITION PLAN—A KEY COMPONENT OF ADOLESCENCE FOR YOUR CHILD WITH AUTISM

Adolescence can be a time of storm and stress, but one that can be weathered with a targeted focus on social skills, some preplanning and executive functioning tips, and straightforward, clear communication. However, you need to take the critical action step of developing a transition plan. You want to have that plan in place prior to adulthood, so start working on it while your child is still in the early years of adolescence.

> A well-thought-out, person-centered transition plan is key to your teen's success in moving into adulthood.

The checklist on page 233 is a tool for developing your plan and keeping track of progress.

Steps You Can Take to Promote Healthy Sexuality in Your Teen

1. Communication. Establish a safe opportunity to have a dialogue about sexuality.

2. Sexual education. Ensure that your child receives formal sexual education.

3. Take seriously questions about sexual identity. Be open and aware that your child has a higher than average likelihood of having a diverse sexual orientation or gender dysphoria and provide an environment for your child that supports this.

4. Provide special attention for girls. The research suggests that females with autism are engaging in more sexual behavior than their male peers despite lower reported sexual drive and interest. This mismatch suggests that our female teens and adults with autism have a greater vulnerability with regard to achieving healthy sexual relationships. We've already discussed challenges in understanding and using social cues to guide healthy behavior and having fewer peer relationships to practice social interactions, so it makes sense that choosing romantic partners and avoiding unhealthy sexual relationships will be difficult for both girls and boys with autism. Additionally, new research on girls with autism suggests that girls tend to use social scripts more than boys to guide their social behavior. Unfortunately, there are few social scripts for appropriate private sexual behavior in our culture, leaving our teenage and adult females with autism without a key crutch for engaging with the social world. So, for your female teenager with autism, we reemphasize the critical need for communication and appropriate sexual education but also recommend that you provide concrete social scripts regarding appropriate sexual and romantic behavior, which will help guide your daughter's behavior and promote healthy sexual and romantic choices.

Adult Transition Checklist

The following checklist outlines the steps you will want to take to establish your transition plan and to help track your steps to success. As you collaboratively work through the steps to success with your transition team, you will want to establish a timeline for your key processes and complete any necessary applications (for funding, housing, etc.) in the appropriate time frame.

Activity	Learn more	Put in place/ apply	Questions	To do	Due date	Done
Evaluate your goals and your child's goals						
Establish your transition team						
Draft your child's profile						
State developmental disability agency						
Supplemental Security Income						
Medicaid						
Guardianship						
Financial planning/trust						
Education						
Employment						
Day program/ community engagement						
Residential support/ housing						
Healthcare (primary care provider, psychiatry, other)						
Voter registration						
Selective Service registration						
Advocacy						
Transportation						

Retrospective parent interviews all highlight effective transition planning as the key factor in adult success. This makes sense given that science tells us that the best predictors of success in adulthood for individuals with autism are improved social skills, the identification of goals and development of self-advocacy skills, strong collaborative supports in place, and an understanding of career options. These components of a strong transition plan are all described below.

As you did when your child's original treatment plan was designed, for this transition plan you will assemble your team, you'll marshal your resources, and you'll forge a path that is specific to your child's needs and strengths. It may seem overwhelming to have to do this again. "Wait, what? I'm getting ready to start breathing a little easier as a parent!!" You may see other parents have more free time as their children gain more independence. Just like when you started your treatment team, you'll want to muster supports for yourself and make sure you're taking care of yourself by using the same tools described in Chapter 5 (also see the box on the facing page).

The transition plan is going to look different for each individual, much like the unique treatment plan you established when your child was first diagnosed. Consider the following three points to ensure that the transition plan is a good fit for your individual teen: What are your child's goals? Who should be on the transition team? What supports do you need to put in place?

What Are Your Child's Goals?

Think about your child's goals and also your goals for your child. One way to think about this question is to have the transition plan team ask: Is the target to support independent living or to support lifelong learning but not necessarily independence? Some teens with autism may successfully live independently as adults, and the transition plan can include steps to take to achieve that goal. Others may not be able to develop the skills to live independently, so the transition plan will focus on how to help your child live the fullest life that he can live with as much independence as possible.

The factors that will come into this decision making include the degree of your child's core autism challenges (communication ability,

The Transition Age and Your Own Self-Care

Transition is a process, and it can be stressful. In fact, it may seem as stressful as the time after you first received your child's diagnosis and began activating your resources and pulling together a road map for your child's treatment plan. Here are a few questions to ask yourself and a few suggestions to help guide how you're going to take care of yourself during this transition process.

1. What are your ideas about what disability is? Do you hold assumptions about what disability means for your child's life as an adult? Clarify your principles and explore your own assumptions around disability.

2. What are the short- and long-term goals that you have defined as a caregiver, and what are your child's short- and long-term goals? Break the goals down in terms of a timeline.

3. Let your principles (and not your assumptions) and your and your child's goals drive your actions.

4. Realize what things you have control over and which you don't. Ignore the ones over which you have no control.

5. Plan what steps you need to take to reach your goals and write them down. These steps are the framework of your transition plan.

6. Finally, find like-minded people who share your principles and who have the same goals. They will be a marvelous support for you.

social skills, restricted and repetitive patterns of behavior), cognitive ability (IQ), behavioral disturbances, mental health problems (e.g., anxiety, depression), medical problems (e.g., epilepsy, sleep problems), adaptive skills (self-care, life skills), and access to supportive services (e.g., case management or community support). For some children, determining the appropriate target can be an easy process; for other children it may not be so easy to determine what is most appropriate. This is a tough question to ask as a parent. For some parents it may be easy to identify the appropriate target, yet hard to come to terms with. If you're in that camp, you're not alone. One of the most common fears we hear from parents whose children seem unlikely to live independently involves what their children will do when they are no longer able to take care of them. This may be almost a universal fear for parents of youth with autism. That fear can get in the way of choosing the appropriate target, so an honest appraisal based on the challenges your child may or may not have will help you and the transition team determine the appropriate target.

As part of transition planning it is important to develop your child's personal profile. This profile will include your child's personal life story highlighting important events and relationships and other aspects of your child's life that have helped shape her. This helps set the stage for identifying the personal preferences, strengths, and interests of your child. Identifying critical life events and relationships helps to make sure that none of your child's interests and preferences are left out. Sometimes it's difficult for children with autism to identify goals, dreams, and preferences, so developing your child's profile helps your team fill in those missing pieces. During your transition planning meeting you will then review your child's personal profile, discuss your child's current environment, brainstorm visions for the future, identify obstacles and opportunities, and identify strategies and discuss short-term action steps.

Who Should Be on the Transition Team?

You'll want to assemble a team of individuals engaged and involved with your teenager. Just as in the treatment team planning you did when your child was diagnosed, this process involves a team of people who care about your child, working together to help him move forward to reach his goals. This team would include your child, you, other engaged caregivers, your child's teacher, and, depending on your target, may include a school psychologist, an employment expert, a case manager at a state developmental disabilities agency, or a vocational rehabilitation counselor. You'll want to include individuals who can identify the unique challenges your child faces to ensure these will be addressed.

Your child is the key person on your transition team. A person-centered planning approach ensures that the plan has your soon-to-be-an-adult child's goals at the center of the target. A person-centered planning approach includes your child fully, helps to uncover how she wants to live her life, and identifies what supports are needed to help create a meaningful and productive life. Your person-centered transition team should meet regularly to discuss progress and identify strategies to reach those goals, and everyone on the team should take action to make sure that strategies discussed in meetings are implemented. There are some helpful websites on transition planning you might consult; see the Resources at the back of the book.

What Supports Do You Need to Put in Place?

Identifying or creating natural supports will be a key component of your transition plan, and science suggests that a strong, supportive community combats isolation and the development and exacerbation of mental health concerns while bolstering development and growth. You can imagine these supports forming four concentric circles with individuals in each circle who can help support your child and promote her ability to reach her goals (see the diagram on the following page). Of course, the person-centered planning approach you've taken to identify your child's targets and goals will make it clear what supports you will need for your child.

The federal laws about education provide key supports you can take advantage of for your transition-age child during the teen and young adult years. The Individuals with Disabilities Education Act (IDEA) mandates the right to public education for all eligible children ages 3–21 years, and IDEA makes schools responsible for providing the supports and services that allow this to happen. That means your child with ASD may qualify for special education services through age 21. One goal of the public education supported by the IDEA is for students to be prepared for employment and independent living when they graduate. That means, depending on your child's transition plan, this preparation process can be a key part of your child's educational program. IDEA requirements are generally facilitated through the IEP process, which must include transition planning for all special education students by age 16; see the box on page 239.

To determine if your child should be given a diploma prior to age 21, your child's IEP team may not rely solely upon whether she has completed the sufficient number of credits and coursework for graduation. The team must also consider whether your child is prepared for further education, employment, and/or independent living. Your child's IEP team

The CIRCLE OF INTIMACY. Comprised of people with whom your child shares deep secrets and sincere emotions. These are people (maybe pets or objects) that are valued and dear to your child. This could include family members or not.

The CIRCLE OF FRIENDSHIP. This includes friends or relatives who your child participates in activities with (e.g., goes to dinner, sees a movie), but not those held to the same level of intimacy.

The CIRCLE OF PARTICIPATION. This is where natural supports will be found. This could contain spiritual groups, places of employment, where your child went or goes to school, clubs, organizations, athletic teams, or anywhere else you participate and interact with people.

The CIRCLE OF EXCHANGE. This is where people who are paid to be in our lives reside. This includes doctors, teachers, dentists, social workers, therapists, etc.

What Should Be Included in Your Teen's Transition IEP?

The goal of special education services is to provide students with the transferable skills, competencies, and real-life experiences necessary to excel during and after high school, such as in an employment or a higher education setting. This means that your transition IEP will include:

- A description of your child's strengths and present levels of academic achievement and functional performance
- Measurable postsecondary education goals
- Corresponding IEP goals that enable the student to meet postsecondary education goals
- Clearly stated descriptions of the transition services needed
- A timeline for achieving goals
- The identified responsible people or agencies to help with those goals
- Clarification of how those roles will be coordinated
- A plan for identifying postgraduation services and supports and obtaining the necessary funding to access them

must consider whether her transition goals have been met and whether there is a need for continued transition services to help her achieve the desired goal upon graduation. The team then must identify the services needed to achieve that goal. It's possible for a student to earn enough credits to graduate but not have met his IEP goals related to transition. In such situations, the student should remain in school. Sometimes disputes arise about this. If there is a dispute about whether the transition plan is appropriate or whether your child should receive a diploma, you may file for mediation and due-process proceedings as outlined in the IDEA law.

This educational transition plan is important to put in place during your child's teenage years because all the legal rights that you as parents have regarding special education services for your child are turned over to your child at age 18. If a guardian has been appointed prior to age 18, then the guardian retains the rights, not the student. However, a student who is his own legal guardian may be identified as unable to provide consent for his own education, so there is a process in place for parents to maintain a decision-making role even if a student maintains legal guardianship over his education. In the next chapter, we'll provide information about guardianship and other legal issues about adulthood.

Remember, each family and individual who transitions into adulthood will take a different path. Some teens may graduate high school and move on to postsecondary education. Some may pursue employment and live independently. Others may remain living at home or move into a supported living situation and require more substantial daily support. Each path will be unique. But by educating yourself about the key components, such as employment, housing, finances, and legal considerations, you can develop a meaningful transition plan and use that to guide the process as your child crosses the threshold into adulthood. The following chapter will focus on how to support your adult with autism across the various domains of postsecondary education, employment, housing, mental health issues, guardianship, finances, and self-care.

◈

Take-Home Points

- Teens with ASD encounter a host of new situations and new demands on their less highly developed social skills. They need lots of support from parents, educators, clinicians, and peers at this stage of life.

- Sexuality has too often been ignored in autism. Fortunately, this is changing, and sex education programs designed specifically for teens on the spectrum are being developed. It's important to protect the safety and emotional and physical health of teens with ASD, who struggle more than other teens, especially girls with ASD.

- Now is the time to work hard on your child's ability to complete daily routines and functions that are necessary for any degree of independence in adulthood, from household chores to personal hygiene to managing work, transportation, and housing. Look for opportunities to practice such skills while your son or daughter is still a minor.

- As your teen approaches adulthood, it's essential to set realistic goals together and plan for them step by step, using all the resources at your disposal. Research has found that a transition plan is key to a successful adulthood for those with autism.

10

ADULTHOOD AND AUTISM

Let's take a moment to review what we know about what happens when children with autism grow into adults. A recent systematic review of 25 studies following children diagnosed with autism during childhood and then into adulthood suggests that social functioning, cognitive skills, and language abilities remain relatively stable, with some exceptions showing loss of previously attained skills (perhaps because supports and therapy have been removed) and some individuals continuing to gain new skills. The picture looks brighter for adaptive functioning, those everyday skills we use to be independent. These tend to improve for most individuals as they become adults. This means the prognosis for independent or semi-independent functioning is better for many individuals than we thought. Also encouraging is that, while most children maintain the diagnosis of ASD into adulthood, the severity of autism-related symptoms often improves. Core challenges in social communication and repetitive and restricted behaviors tend to decrease as individuals become adults. Across all studies, mental health concerns, such as anxiety and depression, were found to be common, persisting into adulthood and tending to worsen if the adults are isolated. One important conclusion of this review is that inclusion in the community, rather than isolation, is paramount.

The data also tell us that although there is a clear recognition that individuals with autism can make substantial and meaningful contributions in the workplace, adults with autism are employed far less frequently and consistently than adults without autism. Rates of employment vary by study, but researchers have consistently found that only a little over half of adults with autism have held a job and fewer than 25% have full-time work. Generally, adults with autism work fewer hours and receive lower rates of pay than coworkers and tend to have jobs below their skill level.

Housing goes hand in hand with employment. The data regarding housing also tell a sobering story. Although findings vary by study, generally speaking, fewer than a third of adults with autism live independently in their own home. Around 20% live at home with their parents, while about half are living in a shared living situation with a roommate or housemates. The remainder of adults with autism are living in a range of licensed agencies, residential facilities, or group homes. The top concerns about living on one's one, from the perspective of adults with autism, focus on the ability to pay for housing. The fear of isolation, of having inadequate support or continued care from family, are all in distant second place relative to the financial fears associated with living on their own.

While these survey data paint a challenging picture for adulthood, the findings are not all discouraging. First of all, keep in mind that the adult outcomes in this review are for adults who received their diagnosis and initial treatment 15–30 years ago. Our ability to diagnosis and provide appropriate intervention for individuals on the autism spectrum has substantially changed over the past few decades. We would anticipate that the adult outcomes of people who are children now will be much better. Second, the data suggest that outcomes for autism in adulthood are going in the right direction. Employment opportunities are increasing, and increasing numbers of providers are developing expertise and experience in working with adults with autism to address their mental health concerns. Postsecondary education programs are expanding to support success for individuals with autism in academic programs.

> *Independence does not come easily to adults on the spectrum, but many are more independent today than we used to think was possible, and many keep gaining adaptive skills as they age.*

Novel housing opportunities promote independence. These developments mean that resources are increasingly available to support your adult child's ability to continue learning, to gain skills, and to continue to be a vital, included part of the community and achieve her goals.

HOW CAN YOU HELP YOUR YOUNG ADULT SUCCEED?

Let's review the important to-dos to promote success for your adult child with autism, whether that be concerning postsecondary education, employment, housing, medical and mental health care, or financial and guardianship information.

Postsecondary Education

While education after high school is not the right fit for every child, it may be the appropriate target for your child. If a focus on postsecondary education is one of your child's goals and the transition team that you've assembled is aligned with this target, a range of postsecondary education options is available. We can break these opportunities down into three main types: mixed/hybrid models, substantially separate models, and inclusive individual-support models.

In the *mixed/hybrid* model, students with ASD participate in social activities and/or academic classes with students who don't have disabilities. The curricula at times are augmented with classes focused on building adaptive skills, sometimes referred to as "life skills" or "transition" classes. This model typically provides students with supported employment experience either on or off campus.

In the *substantially separate* model, your young adult with ASD would participate only in classes with other students with disabilities. These classes are sometimes referred to as part of a "life skills" or "transition" program. In these models, students may have the opportunity to participate in social activities on campus and may be offered employment experience. The employment opportunities are often through a rotation of preestablished employment slots either on or off campus.

In the *inclusive individual-support* model, students receive individualized services to support success in college courses, certificate programs, and/or degree programs. The courses and programs can be taken for credit or can be audited if college course work credit is not needed. The specialized services can range from support through an educational coach or tutor to additional supports through technology or naturalistic supports like those your student may have received as part of a 504 plan in high school. Your child's vision, career goals, and unique needs would drive the selection of services. The focus of this type of program is on establishing a student-identified career goal that directs her course of study and employment experiences. Those practical, supervised employment experiences could include internships, apprenticeships, or other work-based learning opportunities.

If you and your child are considering postsecondary education, it's important to note that having an IEP or 504 plan does not automatically result in accommodations for college entrance exams, such as the SAT, ACT, or Advanced Placement exams. So it's important to know what is involved in requesting accommodations for these types of tests. Usually you can work with your child's school to submit the accommodation requests, but you can submit a request directly without the school's involvement if you prefer. The review process can take up to 2 months, so make sure to plan ahead. Information about the College Board exams and the materials for accommodation requests for students with disabilities is available online at *http://student.collegeboard.org/services-for-students-with-disabilities*.

Other critical information to consider is that your child's IEP from high school does not extend into postsecondary education. Section 504 of the Rehabilitation Act of 1973, which prohibits discrimination based upon disability, provides protections for a "qualified individual with a disability," as does the Americans with Disabilities Act, but "qualified" is a key piece of that sentence. In this instance, "qualified" means your child is capable of fulfilling the essential functions and requirements of the program, with or without "reasonable modifications." So, there is some gray area there, but just as when you established your IEP for your child, communicating with the various professionals involved in your life and providing the necessary information to your child's team will ensure that

> *Postsecondary accommodations and educational programs don't automatically follow from the supports your child received in high school, so be sure to think ahead; applying and obtaining what your child needs to succeed in higher education can take time.*

the reasonable modifications can be identified. Importantly, in postsecondary education, to receive accommodations, your child must identify himself as having a disability, and you will have to specifically request accommodations. This may prove problematic for some of you who do not wish to label your child as a person with disabilities in the college setting. However, this is a requirement to request accommodations on all campuses that provide services.

That may seem like a lot to sift through, but there are also resources in the community to help you navigate the complexities of postsecondary education for your child with autism. There are private consulting companies that assist families with autism in specialized college counseling or employment readiness, such as building skills for interviewing and on-the-job skills. These types of programs help students with autism and their families navigate the available college options prior to applying, during the application, and during college. Additionally, the many postsecondary institutions around the country can provide assistance navigating the range of training and certification programs and individualized and group support services that are available. And more programs and services are being developed as we write this.

Employment

There are several factors that can help an adult with ASD be more successful in obtaining and keeping a job. These include learning to be more independent (e.g., time management, personal care, meal preparation) and avoiding social isolation (i.e., engaging in frequent activities outside the home where one can learn to adjust to new environments and interact with others). Also, when an adult is struggling with anxiety and/or depression, it is important that the person get help, since mental health problems can interfere with an adult's ability to function well in a workplace environment. As we mentioned earlier, anxiety and depression are common in adolescents and adults with ASD. There are also well-established treatments for these conditions, through both behavioral intervention and medicines. So seeking treatment is important for best outcomes for adults on the autism spectrum. Science also tells us that there are many other variables that predict successful employment (see the box on the following page). Some of them you can't control, but others you can, such as establishing a strong transition plan that engages your child's high school in working with the community to support placement after high school.

What Science Tells Us Are Some of the Best Predictors of Successful Employment for Adults with Autism That You Can Influence

- Better daily living (adaptive skills)

- Social skills

- Receiving career counseling in high school

- Transition planning, including job experience while in high school

- Contact by the high school with postsecondary vocational training programs or potential employers

- Matching interests, skills, and strengths of each person with a particular job

- Job coaching on interview skills

- Training and coaching opportunities related to specific skills needed for the job

- Availability of job mentors

- Training of employers on the unique needs of people with autism

- Willingness of the employer to provide environmental supports, such as changing the lighting or sound in the work environment

The next section describes some of the ways you can help your child prepare for employment success.

It's All about Preparation

Preparing to help your child succeed at work includes exploring career options. Finding a good match is key to your child's successful employment. He can explore career options by volunteering at different places, getting an internship, or job shadowing. This of course requires effort and collaboration between families, schools, and employers.

Educate yourself about the different types of employment opportunities:

- First, there is *competitive employment*. This would be a full- or part-time paying job where usually no long-term support is provided.

• *Supported employment* involves work in competitive jobs in which the individual receives ongoing support while on the job. The amount of supervision may be decreased over time as the person learns tasks associated with the job. This type of employment is usually funded through vocational rehabilitation agencies or state developmental disabilities agencies. For this type of employment, you will likely have to advocate strongly. By definition supported employment is intended for individuals with severe disabilities, and funding is often limited.

• In *customized employment* job tasks or duties are negotiated with businesses based on finding creative ways to identify and use the strengths and abilities of the individual with autism. In this type of employment structure a unique relationship between the employer and employee is established. There are few organizations that facilitate this type of arrangement, so it will also likely require advocacy and work from members of your child's transition team to get this process started as your child transitions into adulthood.

• Finally, *sheltered employment* programs are those in a protected environment that provides training and services to assist adults with autism in developing life skills as well as educational and prevocational skills. Again, these models are usually supported by state programs and subject to funding.

One young woman with autism whom one of us (Bernier) worked with, Suzanne, had an entrepreneurial mother who was very actively engaged in the community as a member of the chamber of commerce. Suzanne's mother reached out to several area businesses to advocate for her daughter with autism. She highlighted her daughter's meticulous attention to detail, strict adherence to rules and regulations (she used the word strict in place of "rigid," which may have been more accurate), and consistent timeliness to highlight how productive her daughter would be in a business environment that did not require significant social interaction. By doing this, Suzanne's mother facilitated a customized employment position for her daughter, who has been happily working in the same setting for 6 years.

Aside from acquiring information about employment, it's important to check your own assumptions or messages you hear from others.

I worked with one mother who heard from her child's school counselor that her child's self-worth was connected to employment—that Joe, her child, would not be whole if he were not employed. However, there are very many happy people—with and without autism—who do not "work" for a paycheck but have a meaningful life through community involvement or work that is not typical. It's critical that we rethink how we view employment so that it is not just about receiving a paycheck but about contributing to society in a way that engages with the community. It all relates to the person-centered planning in the type of transition plan discussed in Chapter 9. Joe's mom worked with his department of vocational rehabilitation case manager to find a great position for Joe volunteering at a children's hospital clinic, where he performed a number of supportive tasks (e.g., cleaning toys and testing materials, supporting clinic team-building activities, filing medical records). He was not earning a paycheck but was meaningfully contributing and engaged with a variety of individuals and reported being very happy in this placement. The goal in this case was to allow Joe to gain skills in a work setting, even if only on a volunteer basis. Down the road, Joe can use the skills and experience he gained volunteering to apply for a paid job, if he wishes to do so.

Joe's story is a good example of job matching. Joe's cognitive impairments and challenges with organization and time management, along with significant social deficits, made it difficult for him to initially succeed in competitive employment. He was not motivated by money but was motivated by his ability to help others and share sports facts and information with others. A volunteer position in an environment with flexible coworkers with a high level of education about autism and an onsite employee who could manage Joe's time for him was the perfect job match. And it turns out that the science on employment in autism suggests that the most important consideration in helping your adult child with autism find a job is the job match.

When helping your child find a good job match, three broad areas must be considered: (1) your child's interests, motivation, and skills; (2) your child's learning style; and (3) the environmental demands, such as the communication, sensory, social, and organizational demands. Assessing the motivating factor is also critical, and again you can fall back on the person-centered plan you have developed, because many individuals with autism are not motivated by money. Your adult child's motivation to work will be directly related to how much he enjoys the work he is being asked to do. When considering job options it will be important to assess for both the physical components (hours of employment, pay, leave, benefits, acceptable margin of error, production requirements, physical requirements, etc.) and the social components (clear job expectations, acceptable level of interaction with coworkers/supervisors, demands on communication skills, coworker training and support). Both physical and social demands will contribute significantly to the job match.

Importantly, both Suzanne and Joe found meaningful work, and despite significant social and behavioral challenges associated with their autism diagnosis, they were able to maintain lasting, successful jobs because of successful job matching, thanks to parental preparation, identification of key target goals through a strong transition plan, and an understanding of their motivation and skills and the demands of the job.

Day programs are available that can help promote inclusion in the community for individuals who are not able to function in a paid work setting. Day programs provide structured activities and specialized supports that allow individuals with autism to participate in non-employment-related activities on-site and in the community. These programs can be paid for privately, with state-supported respite dollars or

Job matching has been shown in research to be critical to success in the workplace for adults with autism. The match needs to take into account not just the prospective employee's abilities but also what the adult with ASD really likes and wants to do in a job.

Another key factor for success in employment is to find an employer who recognizes the skills and benefits that people with autism bring to the workplace and who is willing to provide the necessary supports that are required for success. These include (1) recognition that people with ASD are not likely not going to be highly skilled at conducting a typical interview, which requires a considerable level of social skills, (2) modifying the work environment, such as the format of the task, lighting, and sound levels, and (3) availability of a job coach and/or mentor to whom the adult with ASD can turn for training and support.

with Medicaid personal care dollars, depending on what type of contracts the agency that runs the day program has. Many of the day programs require participants to bring a caregiver along if they are not independent in self-help skills (feeding, toileting, etc.). Across the day programs, parents enroll their child in the program/activities, provide transportation to and from the program (privately or via public options), and arrange for a caregiver if required.

> Even for those who can't be employed, it's important to have community involvement and structured activities. Preventing isolation through the use of day programs helps to prevent anxiety and depression among adults with autism.

The diagram on the facing page summarizes different approaches to maintaining engagement in the community for adults.

Housing

Housing is another critical component of adult life for your child with autism. As we mentioned at the start of this chapter, the literature states that adults with autism are living in a number of settings ranging from independent housing to residential programs and everything in between. The table on the facing page lists several housing options that are available to your child, and it is important to determine which model is right for you.

Residential options for adults with ASD vary by area, but they generally include: 1) continuing to live at home or residing in a 2) shared living situation, 3) in creative housing solutions, or 4) in an adult family home, group home, or assisted living situation.

Continuing to live at home works marvelously for some families. It means increased time spent with the family and a familiar setting where your child may feel most comfortable and be most successful. Provided it works for everyone in the family and aligns with the goals of your child's transition plan, this may be the most appropriate fit. For an individual whose stated goal is to live independently, living at home may be a temporary phase as all the other pieces are put in place to support successful living outside the family home.

Staff support is provided in shared living housing scenarios, including

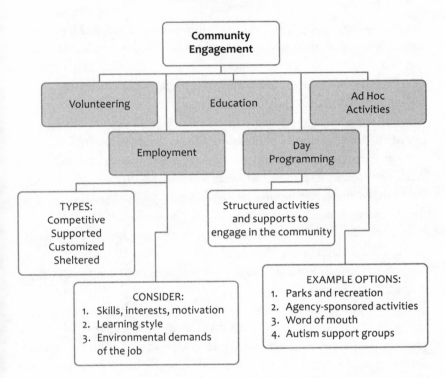

Possible housing options	Potential benefits	Potential drawbacks
Living at home	Increases time spent with family. Familiarity for individual.	May not align if target is independent living.
Shared living situation	Provides staff support.	Costs associated with staffing.
Creative housing situations	Uniquely meet individual's needs, interests, and goals.	Difficult to find or develop.
Assisted living situation	Professional staff support. Availability of peers.	Costs. Less oversight of staffing and individual.
Group home setting	Professional and institutional support. Availability of peers.	Costs. Less oversight of staffing and individual.

the family home or a home the individual rents or owns. Funding for shared living scenarios can come from Section 8 (see below) or other state funding, and caregivers can be hired either by residents or parents.

Creative housing scenarios refer to several different approaches to managing housing, such as sharing an apartment with a roommate who provides support in exchange for reduced rent. Online matching programs support these types of programs. Other creative housing situations include settings such as a farmstead—a working farm for adults with disabilities found in some rural areas or larger residential care facilities. Backyard cottages, mother-in-law-type units in the backyard, are becoming increasingly popular in urban settings for families that can afford to have their adult child continue to live at home, but with more independence. Pocket neighborhoods, which are not disability specific, but can be inclusive and diverse, are small groups of houses or apartments gathered around a shared open space.

Other living arrangements include adult family homes or assisted living in which several individuals with autism live together in a home provided and staffed by a disability agency or in group homes that are similar to adult family homes but offer a higher level of support and higher staff to resident ratio.

Many families rely on government Medicaid waivers or other programs to pay for adult services, including residential support staff for some of these housing options. The federal government adopted the waiver in 1981 so states could pay for residential and other services in communities, rather than for institutions. With federal oversight, states create their own waiver rules. States generally require adults to have a specific disability, a demonstrated need for support services, and financial need. Many services are available only to people who need the high level of care typically found in group home or institutional living situations. Section 8 is a federal housing subsidy allocated by the Department of Housing and Urban Development (HUD) through local housing authorities. Recipients of Section 8 vouchers pay between 30 and 40% of their income toward rent and utilities. The housing authority pays the rest up to a payment standard set by HUD. The recipient can use this voucher to rent from any private-market landlord who accepts Section 8 vouchers. Recipients can keep their voucher as long as they continue to qualify, and it is applicable anywhere in the United States. Section 8 has very long wait lists, so it is important to apply right when your child turns 18 if you are interested in accessing this support system. Applicants are selected using a lottery drawing, and it is possible to apply to multiple waiting lists in different counties and states if your child is flexible in terms of where she will live.

If your adult child with autism is going to be living outside of your home, but not independently, such as in a supported living situation, there are situations you want to avoid to ensure that your adult with autism is safe:

1. A lack of privacy and dignity for the resident

2. An expectation of complete compliance as a condition of residence

3. A high client-to-staff ratio, which limits supervision and opportunities for disclosure

4. Staff without a positive attitude toward the residents

5. Institutional settings that cluster vulnerable individuals together with individuals who are potentially abusive or sexually aggressive

6. Loose standards for "therapeutic restraints"

You should feel entitled to ask questions of the staff for any agency-supported housing situation. You want to make sure these scenarios do not develop. If your child is minimally verbal, it will be especially important for you to keep an eye out for them, as she may not be able to communicate some of these situations to you. The way to do that is to be vigilant, avoid the conditions listed above, stay engaged with your adult child, and watch for behavioral changes, such as increased irritability, disruptive behavior, withdrawal, or changes in eating, sleeping, and self-care. The presence of those behavioral changes warrants more in-depth understanding of the situation.

Other things that you can do to ensure your child has a safe living environment include supporting him in finding activities he enjoys

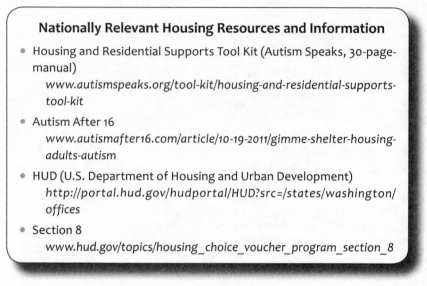

Nationally Relevant Housing Resources and Information

- Housing and Residential Supports Tool Kit (Autism Speaks, 30-page-manual)
  www.autismspeaks.org/tool-kit/housing-and-residential-supports-tool-kit

- Autism After 16
  www.autismafter16.com/article/10-19-2011/gimme-shelter-housing-adults-autism

- HUD (U.S. Department of Housing and Urban Development)
  http://portal.hud.gov/hudportal/HUD?src=/states/washington/offices

- Section 8
  www.hud.gov/topics/housing_choice_voucher_program_section_8

that can boost his self-esteem and being available to talk in a relaxed manner with your child on a regular basis. As we discussed regarding the development of your child's sexuality during the teenage years, open communication is the most important pathway and remains so during the adult years. You can teach your child that there are situations when noncompliance with caregivers is appropriate, such as when a caregiver is being abusive or sexually inappropriate. You can provide support for positive, healthy relationships with romantic partners, which again is modeled through open lines of communication. In terms of the specific housing environment within program facilities, you can make sure a facility carefully screens all staff before employment, choose a facility that supports regular visits by outside client advocacy groups, and be certain that appropriate sexual health education is taught by the program.

Housing options can seem overwhelming, difficult to manage, and terrifyingly expensive—yet you can do it. Many families do. But by educating yourself about the options, identifying your and your child's housing goals, and working with the transition team to put steps in place to achieve that goal, you can find a successful housing scenario for your child. Additionally, many resources are available. The box above contains links to some key national organizations that can help provide information and guidance regarding housing for your adult with autism.

Health Care

When your child transitions into adulthood, she will transition to the adult health care system. Her health care may include both specialty care (specific to autism or to other medical conditions your child has, such as seizures) and primary/preventive care. This transition will be beneficial because your child will receive appropriate screening for and treatment of adult health problems, have access to adult inpatient services and subspecialties (like neurology), and can access sexuality, fertility, and reproductive health services.

You will have to make some adjustments to adapt to this style of health care for your child. For example, your child's pediatric provider was likely family centered, developmentally oriented (considering school and life progress), and interdisciplinary (meaning your provider will synthesize services from across disciplines into a single access point). Your child's pediatric provider also likely involved you in your child's care in terms of both participation and consent. As your child transitions to adult health care, her adult provider will likely provide more individually based (rather than family centered) care with a more disease-oriented focus, will be multidisciplinary (meaning different providers will provide different services for your adult child), and, without initial input from you, will expect your child to be autonomous and function independently.

A strong health care transition promotes continuity of care for your child's autism-related challenges and establishes the health care team before any crises begin. That way, if there are any crises, the professionals are already part of your child's team and can help support your child most

---

What to Look For in an Adult Health Care Provider

Seek out someone who has:

- A comprehensive approach to assessment and planning
- A willingness to acquire expertise when needed to manage the individual's health care and transition to adult health care
- A readiness to work collaboratively and resolve differences
- A patient-centered philosophy of care

effectively. The ideal health care transition ensures that an adult health care provider is identified and that there is a written health care transition plan with a continuously current medical summary. That medical summary should include information regarding your child's functional and neurological status and cognitive status, including formal test results. This would be information such as IQ scores and information about seizure history, language, and adaptive functioning. The medical summary should note any condition-specific treatment plans and contacts, such as treatments specific to gastrointestinal diagnoses. The summary should also include your child's "health education history" and his understanding of his condition and treatments. That is, what does your adult child know and understand about his autism diagnosis and any other diagnoses that he has? The medical summary should also include a current understanding of prognosis, including effects on reproduction potential, and genetic information, such as the presence of any identifiable and relevant genetic information. Finally the summary should include information regarding self-care needs and information about community resources and support.

Mental health issues are a significant concern for many adults with autism. A recent systematic review found that about 42% of adults with autism experience an anxiety disorder at some point and that about 37% experience a depressive disorder at some time in their life. Given these high rates, vigilance is warranted. It will be important to be alert for symptoms associated with both conditions, along with other mental health conditions. And if you notice any significant change in your adult child's functioning, a visit to your child's provider is warranted. If a mental health provider is already part of your child's treatment team, you can encourage him to have a consultation with that provider. If not, then starting with your child's primary care physician will be a good first step.

Attending to mental health concerns is paramount because these challenges can stand in the way of your adult child's effectively integrating with the community,

> It's important to be alert for anxiety and depression in your adult child because unaddressed mental health problems can be an obstacle to engagement with the community, and isolation can increase mental health problems.

and as we've already discussed, being isolated can increase anxiety and depression, working in a cyclical manner.

The Importance of Community Engagement to Health

Think of community engagement this way: for the first 21 years of your child's life school was the active ingredient of daily activity. If your child is not in postsecondary education or engaged in meaningful work, opportunities to continue learning and engage with the social world become increasingly limited. For all adults, both with and without autism, there are fewer opportunities to meet new people and to spend time with existing friends. But for adults with autism it can be even harder because of less involvement in school and work, decreased social initiation, difficulty planning ahead, issues related to anxiety and sensory sensitivities, and a history of unsuccessful social activities. And the research reflects that. Over half of adults with autism report having no participation in a community outing for 12 months while one-fifth report having no social outings for 12-month periods. Despite these challenges, many (if not most) adults with autism report wanting friends and wanting to socialize. Many adults report feeling lonely, isolated, hopeless. And, given the importance of physical activity for mood, physical health, regulating sleep, and ongoing learning, it's important that adults with autism find groups and organizations that will provide these opportunities and help structure them. Without continued growth and learning, it is easy for depression or anxiety or other mental health concerns to fill the void. Research shows that community inclusion and physical activity combat mental illness, so helping your adult with autism remain engaged in the community is a form of preventive medicine.

You can help promote inclusion and your child's involvement in activities by looking for opportunities sponsored by local parks and recreation departments, local Meetup groups for shared interests, organizations and agencies that support social outings for individuals with autism and other disabilities, or by seeking out opportunities through autism support groups or social media outlets associated with autism. Possibilities can range from participation in a social skills group for adults to involvement in sports or Special Olympics. Or perhaps building on your child's interests you could promote involvement in hikes outdoors, therapeutic riding, art and music, dance, yoga, or martial arts. Or really anything at all that you can think of.

Transportation: A Surmountable Obstacle to Community Engagement

One of the often-overlooked challenges to participating in community activities that many adults face is a lack of independent transportation. But there are ways you can help with transportation. The best way is to teach your adult child how to use public transportation in your area, if available. In cities, there are many services in place that your child can take advantage of. There are reduced-fare permits; there are instruction programs that provide free training services to teach individuals with disabilities how to ride public transit. Some buses and light-rail systems have automated audio and visual stop announcement reader boards inside of the vehicle to let riders know when the bus has reached their stop. External audio announcements inform riders of the approaching bus's route and destination. These are accommodations that can be helpful for some adults with autism. There are also some taxi services that have options to prepurchase taxi vouchers at a significant discount for individuals with disabilities to promote the use of cabs to move through the community. There are lots of options that might require some digging, but a little digging early on can make things a whole lot easier later.

Decision Making

Generally speaking, a youth who turns 18 obtains the right to consent to her own health care, education, and financial decisions. But your child with autism may still need assistance with making decisions about critical choices after she turns 18. Even though your child may have attained a new legal status overnight on her 18th birthday, from a biological perspective there is nothing magical about the 18th birthday. Given that, it may seem odd that you have to get the court's permission to do the things you've always done for your child, but that is the reality once your son or daughter turns 18. Thus, if your child lacks the capacity to understand the risks and benefits of critical life choices like medical treatment, finances, housing, or education, you may need to consider guardianship so that you or another responsible adult can help make those decisions.

Guardianship

Guardianship is a court process that provides substitute decision making in which the guardian makes the decision instead of the "incapacitated person," or "principal," as the person with ASD is described in legalese. Guardianship is the most restrictive option because it *deprives* individuals of the ability to make most decisions. Guardianship is appropriate where the person is incapable of making those decisions and is at risk of being harmed. Guardianship is not appropriate merely because the parent does not like the decisions the youth makes or thinks they are unwise. Limited guardianship is an alternative. This allows guardianship to cover only specific responsibilities, like health care, education, or banking.

There are two types of guardianship: estate and person. The types of decisions associated with guardianship of person include housing, health care, and educational decisions. This would involve things like providing informed consent or making decisions on driving or marriage. The right to vote is not taken away with guardianship. In the case of person guardianship, the court must determine based on presented evidence that the individual is at significant risk of personal harm based upon a demonstrated inability to *adequately provide for nutrition, health, housing, or physical safety.* For estate guardianship, which concerns managing funds, applying for benefits, and entering into contracts, the court must determine that the individual is at significant risk of financial harm based upon a demonstrated inability to *adequately manage property or financial affairs.*

Within both types of guardianship (estate and person), the guardian can have either full or limited guardianship. As its name suggests, "full" grants guardianship over everything within that type (person or estate), while limited guardianship is tailored to fit an individual's needs. For example, limited estate guardianship might include managing a certain amount of money.

The guardianship process is straightforward and follows specific timelines. Before you can file a guardianship request with the court, there is a mandatory training. Filing requires completion of some paperwork along with a fee (or a fee waiver can be requested but must be accompanied by an in-person filing request). Cost for guardianship varies depending on the state and county. At the time of filing the court appoints a

---

Common Questions about Guardianship

- Who can file?
  - The person who files can be the proposed guardian or someone else with an interest in the case
- Where can the case be filed?
  - Superior Court in the county where the child lives (generally)
- How do you get a filing fee waiver?
  - Based on the principal's assets (*not* the parent's assets), depending on state and county
- What are the reporting requirements?
  - There are mandatory 90-day reports
  - There are mandatory annual reports
  - These reports are not difficult but are necessary
  - There are additional reports if also guardian of the estate

---

guardian ad litem (GAL). The GAL speaks to the allegedly incapacitated person and notifies him of his rights, obtains a medical report, and makes a recommendation to the court about whether the person is incapacitated, whether a guardianship is necessary, and what the proposed scope of a guardianship should be. Usually 45–60 days after filing there is a guardianship appointment hearing where the outcome is presented. After being appointed, a guardian must return to court regularly to report on the health and financial status of the individual. A 90-day report is due, and annual reports are due to the court. This process is not complex but does require some care by the guardian to see that it is followed.

You can start the guardianship process around 6 weeks before your child's 18th birthday. You can do so after that as well; coordination with your child's birthday is only needed if there's an upcoming medical issue or decision-making situation that will soon follow your child's birthday.

Power of Attorney

There are also less restrictive alternatives to guardianship, such as a power of attorney. Adults who have the capacity to make decisions and therefore don't need guardianship could use power of attorney as an alternative. This is most appropriate for individuals who are less cognitively impaired because the individual must have the capacity to make decisions but need some help, such as when making important decisions or doing financial planning.

Power of attorney is a legal instrument in which one person grants another person the right to make decisions on her behalf. The individual granting the right has the capacity to do so, and the individual does not lose the right to make decisions. If there is a conflict between the decision of the individual and the person granted the power of attorney, the individual's decision has priority. This means, importantly, that a parent or other person with a power of attorney can't override the adult child's decisions, as a guardian can. A power of attorney can only help you implement decisions that accord with your child's wishes. Also important is that, with a power of attorney, your child is not protected from bad decisions. A power of attorney does not involve the court system. See the table below for a comparison of guardianship and power of attorney.

Other, Less Restrictive Options

In addition to power of attorney, there are some other, less restrictive options. For example, representative payee is an option specifically for individuals who receive benefits administered through the Social Security

Differences between Guardianship and Power of Attorney

	Guardianship	Power of attorney
Capacity	Individual lacks capacity to make decision	Individual has capacity to make decisions
Type of decision making	Substitute decision making	The person who has the power of attorney authority acts as supplemental "helper"
Process	Court process	Notarized document
Starts	Court appoints guardian	With the date written in the power of attorney
Ends	As stated in guardianship order	Written rescission

Administration, such as Supplemental Security Income (SSI; see the section on finances below for further information). The representative payee is an individual designated by the Social Security Administration who can act on behalf of the individual receiving benefits (beneficiary). In this situation, the representative payee receives and handles the SSI benefits and agrees to use the benefits on behalf of the beneficiary for the beneficiary's well-being and personal care.

Finances

Some of the most common questions asked by parents of transition-age youth or adults with autism in my (Bernier's) clinic concern finances: How can we pay for all the intervention services? How can we support our child's financial needs given housing and health care costs? In this section we'll review some of the key resources and options to consider regarding finances and your adult with autism to point you in the right direction and give you the general lay of the land. Consultation with an attorney or financial adviser who has expertise in the laws and financial systems in your state concerning adults with disabilities, however, should inform your planning. So, our first recommendation is to seek out consultation from an attorney or other professional with expertise in this domain. Our second recommendation is to educate yourself on some of the available options. We'll restrict our discussion to those resources that are widely available nationwide, but your state will have specific services, resources, and laws applicable to your family.

We can start with Medicaid. Medicaid is a federal program that helps cover medical costs for people with limited income and is available to individuals with disabilities. There are no premiums, deductibles, or co-pays associated with this coverage. Medicaid also provides coverage for long-term care in the form of personal care or assisted living for eligible individuals. More information about Medicaid is available at *www.medicaid.gov*.

SSI is another federal program that provides financial assistance to individuals with disabilities. Individuals do not have to have a history of employment and can be eligible based on the presence of a disability. To be eligible an individual must not have any "substantial gainful activity," which means that the person cannot earn more than a specific amount of money per month. Individuals accessing SSI can receive funds each month to be used for basic necessities. The monthly amount is reduced by earned or unearned income. If an individual is eligible for SSI and income is received, that individual is automatically eligible for Medicaid.

SSI is available for children with disabilities, but parental income is incorporated into the eligibility criteria for children. If a child receives SSI, the Social Security Administration will start a process of reassessment before the child turns 18, though the review may not be complete by the child's 18th birthday. This reassessment happens automatically, and during that process the child's medical records are reviewed to determine whether the child qualifies under the adult SSI standards. The family will receive notice if SSI is being terminated and there are appeal rights, but that appeal must be submitted right away (within 10 days) for the child to receive continuing benefits.

There are also state-supported programs throughout the country focused on community services for individuals with developmental disabilities. These developmental disability programs provide a range of services, and all have specific stipulated eligibility criteria. When funding is available, these state-sponsored programs generally provide: support for employment and day programs; vocational, employment, and educational assistance; mental health programs; and housing support. Some programs include funding for respite or for services to address challenging behavior. Your state will have specific application procedures and eligibility requirements.

It's important to note that for some benefits, including SSI and Medicaid, having too many assets may disqualify your child for eligibility (employment income or more than $2,000 in assets). However, financial mechanisms can be put in place that allow your child to have assets and not be disqualified from government benefits. A couple of options are special needs trusts and ABLE accounts.

A special needs trust is a specific type of trust set up for an individual with a disability. The "trustee" administers the trust, and the "beneficiary" is the person with disabilities whom the trust is for. A special needs trust serves two main purposes. The first is to provide financial coverage, and the second involves coordination with public benefits. Funds in the special needs trust are used to cover things that SSI and Medicaid do not cover. For example, this could include any medical and dental care that is not covered by government benefits, or costs associated with travel, entertainment, clothing, and education. The use of a trust to maintain assets also ensures that private funds do not take away from public benefits for which your child would otherwise be eligible.

To establish a special needs trust you will need to work with an attorney. We strongly encourage you to consider hiring an attorney who specializes in special needs trusts or estate planning. There is no minimum amount of money necessary to start or maintain a special needs trust. And the trust can be set up with the disabled person's own assets or established by a third party (such as you, as the parent) for the benefit of the disabled person. For example, parents may provide for a special needs trust in their wills to be established with a disabled child as the beneficiary. When the disabled child receives that trust, it will not disqualify her from SSI and Medicaid benefits she may qualify for as an adult. An established special needs trust can be listed as a beneficiary of parents' retirement accounts, life insurance policies, or Social Security survivor benefits, just like an individual may be. Monetary gifts and inheritances from family members and friends, and even deeds to property, can also be held by the trust. However, we want to caution you and state clearly that government benefit rules are subject to change, and the different programs, such as Medicaid and SSI, have different rules with respect to special needs trusts. So it will be important to work closely with your attorney regarding the establishment of such a trust.

ABLE accounts are another financial mechanism to support individuals with disabilities. ABLE accounts are tax-free savings accounts for individuals with disabilities and their families. These accounts were created following passage of the Achieving a Better Life Experience (ABLE) Act of 2014. Contributions to an ABLE savings account, which can be made by any person (e.g., the individual, family, or friends), must be made using post-tax dollars, but any income earned by the accounts will not be taxed. Similar to special needs trusts, assets in an ABLE account do not "count against" an individual for determining eligibility for public benefits that are restricted to individuals with limited assets. These protected accounts were developed based on the recognition of the significant extra costs associated with living with a disability.

The ABLE Act limits eligibility to individuals with a disabling condition that began before their 26th birthday. An individual who is already receiving benefits through SSI is automatically eligible. If the individual is not receiving SSI benefits but has a disability with onset prior to age 26 and a letter from a physician confirming that and meets the SSI criteria regarding significant functional limitations, he or she could still be eligible. If you're interested in establishing an ABLE account, you're not required to work with a financial institution within your state. While that was the original intention of the act, Congress modified it in 2016 so that regardless of where you live and whether or not your state has decided to establish an ABLE program, you are free to enroll in any state's program provided that the program is accepting out-of-state residents. Programs have a $14,000 maximum contribution per year, which can be managed easily through the online portal. Money can be used for "qualified disability expenses," a broad category that can certainly address costs associated with education, housing, transportation, basic living expenses, and health, among others. As with tax-advantaged "state 529" college savings plans, multiple options and varied investment strategies are available with ABLE accounts. Some auditing is required, so it will be helpful for you to keep a logbook with a record of what funds from the ABLE account were spent on or used for. Information regarding ABLE accounts is located online at *www.ablenrc.org.*

SELF-ADVOCACY

An important milestone for adolescents and adults on the spectrum is becoming a self-advocate. This means knowing one's rights as a person with a disability and recognizing that every person contributes positively to society and should have the opportunity to live a life with meaning, purpose, and joy. Research indicates that the development of self-advocacy skills is a powerful predictor of success in adulthood for individuals with autism. Your child can begin practicing self-advocacy in childhood and adolescence by participating in IEP meetings and making requests for appropriate accommodations in the classroom, such as reducing the sound level or needing a break. One of the first steps toward self-advocacy is developing self-respect and self-determinism. You can begin by encouraging your child on the autism spectrum to become aware of both his challenges and his strengths and to realize that every single person has areas in which he excels and areas in which he has difficulty. Appreciating that this diversity actually makes the world more interesting will help your adolescent value her place in the world.

It can be helpful to provide strong role models of adults with ASD who have been successful—people on the spectrum who have found a way of capitalizing on their uniqueness, whether through writing, art, music, or simply being a trusted and loyal friend or employee.

Stephen Shore, an adult on the spectrum, talks about "developing an advocacy plan." When faced with a difficult situation, he recommends the following to others who have autism: (1) assess the situation and realize that it is OK if you need some help (e.g., you can't understand a set of complex verbal instructions); (2) ask for reasonable help ("Can you repeat those instructions slowly?"); (3) thank the person and explain why you need help ("Thanks a lot. I do better when people speak slowly"); and (4) depending on the situation, consider disclosing your disability ("I have autism, and so language is sometimes hard to follow"). The point is that as your child becomes an adult, it will become more and more essential that she know how to self-advocate. You won't always be there to make sure your child gets the help she needs, so these skills will increase the chances that your adult child with autism will be able to get necessary and deserved help and accommodations.

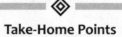

Take-Home Points

- Your adult child should have specific goals for life after high school, preferably set while still in high school. These may include moving right into postsecondary education or employment (paid or unpaid). It's essential to take into account what your son or daughter can and wants to do and to take advantage of all the supports available for reaching those goals.

- It's also important to plan for meaningful community engagement for your child, whether that involves competitive employment, another employment approach, volunteering, or day programming. Avoiding isolation can prevent mental health problems like anxiety or depression.

- Various types of housing arrangements are available, so research what will work best for your adult child.

- Finances always need to be considered. Where applicable, apply for SSI, Medicaid, or state-supported options.

- Many adults with autism need some help with decision making. If your son or daughter is capable of making decisions but needs help, a power of attorney or other less restrictive option may be appropriate. If not, guardianship can protect your child optimally.

Your adult with autism will face a variety of situations that require new skills and support, including finances, employment, housing, and health care concerns. There are a number of steps that you can take to help your child have a successful, meaningful, and productive adult life. The path to this success will start during your child's early teenage years, when you establish a strong transition plan that clearly defines your and your child's goals using a person-centered approach. You and your child will break those goals down into short- and long-term objectives and will tackle them in time. Together you will determine the importance and relevance of postsecondary education, identify the type of community engagement and inclusion that is the best fit, be that employment or other activities, to ensure successful lifelong learning and bolstered mental health. You can help your child establish appropriate adult health care, explore possible housing options, and work with the legal and financial infrastructure to ensure she can access all the available public health benefits and have funds available to meet her needs. The path will likely differ for each family reading this book, but the ultimate end goal will remain the same: for your adult child to lead a happy, healthy, and meaningful life filled with opportunities and hope.

11

TYING IT ALL TOGETHER

In this final chapter we look at a variety of ways that families can use and combine the different kinds of information provided in this book. The best help for individuals with ASD can't be found in one-size-fits-all solutions. Here we aim to help stimulate your own thoughts about what combination of insights might be particularly useful for your son or daughter, your family, and your situation.

For some families, the most important measure to take may involve establishing a strong team and identifying the most appropriate interventions. For others, the focus may be to enhance a healthy lifestyle with diet, exercise, and sleep. For yet another, it may be to support the transition from adolescence into adulthood. Most of you will be best advised to combine these personal steps with professional help. Except for a fortunate few, most lifestyle interventions, like most professional interventions, are only part of the picture.

LIFE ON THE SPECTRUM

As the following stories show, however, the personal steps you take can make the professional help work better and may enable your child to get by with less professional or medical support than otherwise expected—in addition to making your family healthier and easing the burden on all concerned.

Milo: The Role of Self-Advocacy and the Treatment Team

Jessica and Zachary's son Milo is now 9 years old. Their story provides a good example of the self-advocacy and persistence needed in many instances. They were first-time parents who realized something was not quite typical with Milo's development when he was 17 months old. He had been a relatively easy baby—not very fussy, content to sit by himself for extended periods of time, and he started to crawl and then take his first steps at the expected times. However, by a year and half both Jessica and Zachary recognized that he wasn't using any words. When they look back now, they realize that when Milo was in his first year, he didn't look them in the eyes and wasn't as cuddly and affectionate as most babies. Jessica and Zachary just didn't have enough experience to appreciate those subtle signs at the time. During an 18-month-old well-child visit, Milo's pediatrician counseled patience, saying "Some boys talk a little later. Let's see how he does over the next few months." But during the rest of that year, he seemed to do worse, not better. They noticed more unexplainable tantrums and behavioral problems. He seemed to have odd sensory reactions. When he kneeled down and licked the neighbor's doorstep on one afternoon walk 3 months later, Jessica returned to the pediatrician's office.

They wanted to follow the pediatrician's advice and wait, but their instincts told them that a few months was too long to wait. They didn't know anything about autism or what it was, but Jessica asked the pediatrician a lot of questions and pushed to get a further evaluation—an evaluation for what, she did not know, but she knew her son needed an evaluation.

The pediatrician, to his credit, this time placed a referral for evaluation at a specialty autism clinic. (They were fortunate that their community had such a clinic; not all do. However, see our Resources section for opportunities that may be available for low-resource communities.) Here Jessica and Zachary ran into a common problem: They were told that the wait list for an evaluation was several months long. Jessica hung up the phone. But after thinking about it for a little while, she took a deep breath and then called back to ask about cancellations and other evaluation opportunities. The intake worker gave her a list of other clinics in the area and put Milo on the cancellation list. Jessica then got Milo on the wait list for three other area clinics that provided autism evaluations and made a note to call each one frequently to check for cancellations. Then she caught a lucky break, which was available to her because she was able to take off work on short notice—after just 8 days of calling, she was able to take Milo in to one of the clinics for an evaluation the day she called.

At the evaluation Jessica was told Milo had autism. She had a flurry of emotions—an "aha" and validation of her suspicions, mixed with pangs of worry in the pit of her stomach, because she didn't know what to do or to expect.

At first Jessica and Zachary felt numb—both parents felt immediately anxious about their son's future. Would he learn to talk, develop friendships, go to college? Then they shifted back into action. They reached out to the school system and called the providers at the Birth to Three program Milo was in. Jessica contacted a behavioral intervention agency to get a list of all the applied behavioral analysis (ABA) therapists in the community. She pulled together her team and got Milo engaged in behavioral intervention, set up an Individualized Family Service Plan (IFSP; see Chapter 5 regarding IEPs for children under age 3), and devoured as much information about autism as she could. Milo's behavioral plan focused on promoting basic social skills, such as responding to his name, attending to faces, and using and understanding gestures. With that foundation Milo could learn from the rich social environment he was now in and could further his language skills to navigate his social world. Within months, Jessica and Zachary went from feeling helpless to celebrating the new skills that Milo was demonstrating. They also joined a local parent support group for children with autism. Other parents provided helpful advice and emotional support, and new friendships with members of the group were emerging.

Through all of this coordination and planning, Jessica and Zachary made sure to take care of themselves. They made time to be together and share their fears and hopes. Jessica continued with her yoga class, and Zachary still met weekly with a group of friends from work. They learned how to let people know why Milo sometimes behaved differently, explained what autism was to friends and family and sometimes strangers, and were pleased to find that most people were accepting and supportive.

Milo is now in fourth grade, speaking in full sentences, gaining academic skills, and is developing some foundational social skills that he is using with the peers in his regular education classes and with his peers in his special education classes. He continues to benefit from ABA tutoring, speech–language therapy, and occupational therapy. It is fascinating to watch how Milo interacts with the world, and it is clear that, while he has challenges, he has areas of strength as well. He knows the name of every basketball player on the local basketball team, which impresses the other children in his class. Jessica and Zachary are already thinking about how he might use his exceptional memory in a job someday.

Emily and Anna: Different Pictures of Autism

Emily and Anna are nonidentical twins. That is, from a genetic perspective they share the same amount of DNA as nontwin siblings do. They are in sixth grade, and both have a diagnosis of autism. But that is where their similarities end.

Emily and Anna were their parents' first children. The twins were born at 36 weeks via C-section. The family stayed in the hospital for just a couple of days and then went home. Within the first year the twins developed at different rates. Emily's motor skills were delayed. She did not sit up on her own until nearly 10 months, crawled and walked late, and then did not develop single words until after she was 3 years old. Anna's motor development was similar, although she sat up earlier than her sister, but her speech came online around 12 months of age, with phrase speech before she turned 2. While family members told the twins' parents that Anna was just speaking for Emily, the motor concerns pushed them to consult their pediatrician when the girls were around 19 months of age. Emily was finally seen by a developmental pediatrician just before age 3 and diagnosed with autism. At that time Emily was engaging in repetitive motor mannerisms, had difficulties with transitions, had not developed speech, had limited nonverbal behaviors, and showed no interest in other children.

About 2 years after Emily was diagnosed, when the girls were about 5 years old, Emily's early intervention provider suggested that Anna also be evaluated for autism. Emily's provider noticed that although Anna used language, she was mainly sharing facts about things she had read (she was an early reader and devoured facts about animals) or speaking to ask for things. She rarely responded to open-ended prompts, and she neither commented on nor brought up topics related to others' interests or activities. Anna was evaluated and diagnosed with autism at that time.

Now at 12 years old Emily uses phrase speech to communicate, has significant repetitive motor mannerisms (she flaps her hands, lines objects up on the floor, and repeatedly drops things from the same height), and appears to have no interest in her peers or in engaging on a purely social level with her family members. Emily is in a fully contained special education classroom.

Anna, in contrast, is in a regular education classroom and is performing above grade expectations academically. She uses fluent speech, although rarely as part of a social conversation; she mainly uses her language to make requests or share facts about her intense interest in cats. She has an IEP with goals focused on social skills and pragmatic language along with accommodations around sensory aversions—for example, she wears headphones nearly all of the time she is outside her house.

Emily and Anna both have an autism diagnosis, but they have very different manifestations and challenges. Their parents have had to develop individualized plans for both girls. The great differences between these twins illustrates how diverse autism is along its spectrum and how complex the causes of and contributors to autism are.

Billy: The Impact of Associated Challenges

The stories above involved families in big cities with some resources. But many of you are living in places where services for autism are inadequate. This was the case for the Johnson family. Their son, Billy, is now 10 years old. They live in a rural town with limited access to medical providers or health care. Billy was diagnosed at age 5 after he started kindergarten and his parents and teacher noticed that he wasn't making friends or showing interest in peers, he was struggling with transitions in school, and he couldn't manage his behavior in the classroom.

Up until kindergarten Billy was at home most days with his aunt and older sister. Interactions with other children were mostly limited to his sister and their cousins, who lived nearby and with whom they spent time regularly. When the family did go into the community, Billy was with his family and seemed to manage just fine. Looking back with perfect hindsight, Billy's parents recognize that he wasn't very interested in kids he didn't know pretty well, that he wasn't very affectionate or cuddly, and that he seemed to have very intense interests that were the focus of how he spent his time. They did comment on his difficulties with sleep, though they thought this wasn't a big problem. But other than sleep problems, Billy's parents felt that at the time he was doing just fine. But when Billy started school, it became clear that he was having challenges coping with the demands and schedule of the public school setting.

Although the rural community had few resources, Billy's parents were resourceful and worked with the existing resources in the town to support him. They worked with the school to establish an IEP that includes accommodations within his regular education classroom. The school was able to make several adjustments, including social skills instruction, speech therapy, schedule changes, the use of social stories and picture schedules to aid in transitions, a peer buddy system for recess time, and a dedicated quiet space for him near his classroom that he can use if he is struggling. They found a wealth of information through books and reputable organizations online.

While Billy had always struggled with sleep, the impact that his difficulties falling asleep had on him became apparent within the day-to-day parameters of the school schedule. The school psychologist noted during one of the IEP team meetings that Billy often just looked so very tired in the classroom. His parents shared their difficulties with getting Billy into bed and to sleep regularly. They set up a separate meeting to speak in more depth with the school psychologist, where it quickly became clear that good sleep hygiene habits had never been established for Billy, or anyone in the house for that matter.

Billy's parents reported that neither of them had a consistent bedtime routine. Ralph, Billy's father, would fall asleep on the couch watching TV as often as he fell asleep in his bed. Diana, Billy's mother, sometimes stayed up till the wee hours of the morning reading. Both of Billy's parents were big consumers of coffee throughout the day and evening. Neither was physically active; both struggled with their weight. Billy's older sister, Samantha, also had an inconsistent bedtime—she was a bookworm, like her mother, and would stay up quietly in her bed reading.

She did not have any behavioral problems at school, so no one ever commented on her sleep schedule. Billy had no bedtime routine either. There was not a consistent bedtime, there were no routines for Billy, and most of his evening activities, Billy's parents came to learn, actually impeded his ability to fall asleep. He would spend many evening hours after dinner watching movies on the old television in his room. Since one of his favorite activities was bouncing, he would intersperse time jumping on the trampoline in the backyard with his television viewing in the evening. He also loved soda pop and was often rewarded for good behavior with (caffeinated) soda from the nearby convenience store.

The school psychologist, Dr. Singh, provided information about sleep hygiene, referred Billy's parents to some books on sleep habits, and encouraged them to work with Billy's pediatrician around developing healthy sleep hygiene. Ralph and Diana purchased the recommended books (Diana liked to read them late at night) and implemented some basic changes for their family.

It has been over 4 years since Diana and Ralph started working to establish a bedtime routine and promote strong sleep hygiene habits in their home. First they established a strict lights-out bedtime of 9:00 P.M. for Billy. Diana set a timer at 8:30, which indicated it was time for him to brush his teeth and put on pajamas (prior to the implementation of the sleep hygiene program he would often sleep in his clothes). He was allowed to play quietly in his room or read after he brushed his teeth and changed. Then she came to his room to shut the lights off. Diana and Ralph eliminated caffeine from Billy's diet. He is still rewarded with soda, but not caffeinated soda (we'd like to clarify that soda is not healthy for a child Billy's age, and certainly not as frequently as Billy was having it, or as a reward). They removed the old TV from Billy's room so that he could not watch it after dinnertime. Originally they left it in his room and told him he was not to watch TV after 7:00 P.M., but he did not comply with this rule. They also restricted his access to the trampoline after 8:00 P.M. so his "body had time to slow down." It took Billy's mom several months to implement this program, but they had a strong advocate for this in Billy's school principal. Most important, the school team noted a significant improvement in Billy's ability to manage the day-to-day demands in school, and over the years Diana and Ralph were able to reduce their involvement in the bedtime process as the routine became ingrained for Billy. Now, nearly 5 years later, Billy continues to do well at school, and the rest of the family has been sleeping a lot better, too.

Georgia: Understanding and Acceptance as Part of the Narrative

Georgia, now 14 years old, was diagnosed with autism when she was two and half years old. At the time she did not use words to communicate, made no eye contact, had limited facial expressions, and spent the majority of her time waving strings (or anything stringlike) in front of her face. She had macrocephaly (large head circumference), was very tall for her age, had staring spells (which prompted an evaluation by a neurologist, who ended up making the diagnosis), and had significant problems with constipation.

Her parents, Jen and Steven, initially didn't agree with the diagnosis. Jen recalls leaving the appointment and thinking to herself, "How could that neurologist know? He only saw her during that one appointment!" After she cooled off for a couple of days, Jen and Steve did some reading on the Internet, and they realized that Georgia's behavior did suggest a diagnosis of autism. While they followed all the recommendations that the neurologist had listed (e.g., get Georgia involved in behavioral intervention, consult with a gastroenterologist, come in for follow-up seizure evaluations, get involved in a Birth to Three program), Jen found her energy and enthusiasm for life were lagging because she was struggling with depression. After consulting with her primary care physician, she started taking medication for depression and engaged in cognitive-behavioral therapy (CBT), which helped a lot. Her therapist mentioned how important it is to stay connected to other people and not isolate herself. She made time for a weekly gym class and joined a parent support group. With these changes, she felt much more able to take on the challenges ahead.

When she reflects on that "dark year" as she calls it, she remembers worrying about her son, who was only 13 months younger than Georgia. However, Georgia's brother's development progressed normally.

Over the past 10 years Jen has taken Georgia to all of her appointments and diligently worked with the school and the treatment team to support Georgia. There have been few changes in Georgia's language, social abilities, or behaviors during that time, but Jen and her family have changed considerably. Jen made significant efforts to take care of herself. Through Facebook she connected with other parents and began to tell her family's story and hear other stories. She found a community of parents with whom she could share her concerns and her triumphs.

Nowadays Georgia sits at the table with the family every evening for dinner. She doesn't eat the same food, as she has a limited diet, primarily of macaroni and cheese and peanut-butter sandwiches, but she is present. She is involved in every family activity and accompanies the family on all community outings, accompanying her parents on the sidelines of her brother's soccer games. Jen and Steve are both active in her behavioral treatments, and Georgia's 12-year-old younger brother is already a strong advocate for individuals with autism.

Ansel: The Transition to Adulthood

Ansel was diagnosed with autism in the late 1990s when he was 5 years old. As he progressed through school, he developed language, but used words infrequently to communicate. His IEP at school included goals regarding speech, social skills, management of challenging behavior, and adaptive skills. His therapies outside of school included behavioral interventions and medications to help with his challenging behavior. He could become aggressive toward others (familiar individuals and strangers alike), would destroy property (the walls of his house were dotted with holes from kicks and punches), and at times he would bang his head or bite his arm. He made some gains over the course of his elementary and high school life with periodic ups and downs with his challenging behavior.

Ansel was a tall kid and is now a tall, heavyset young man. His size, limited eye contact, limited language, and unpredictable aggressive outbursts pose a serious and worrisome challenge for educators.

Three times in high school he was hospitalized in a psychiatric facility due to unmanageable aggression. The short hospital stays provided limited treatment but did provide respite for his mother, father, and stepfather, who were all actively involved in his life. That respite period was critical for his parents.

During his teenage years, Ansel's parents worked with the school to ensure Ansel could extend his program until he turned 21 (which is an appropriate option for some, as we described in Chapter 9). That provided them more time to consider housing options and programming for the day for Ansel, as he needed continuous supervision and his parents needed to work. Unfortunately, there were times when the school was unable to contain Ansel's challenging behaviors, so alternative coverage was needed on those days when his behavior was unmanageable at school. Ansel's parents worked with their employers to develop flexible work schedules, they contacted state services to request respite, and they called on their extended family to help them manage Ansel's behavior.

Ansel is nearing 21 years old, and his school placement will draw to a close in the spring. His parents are still managing Ansel's behavior through a combination of medication, intermittent behavioral treatments, and the use of respite. The respite care is funded by the state. Ansel's parents also accessed SSI with the help of a social worker and use those funds to support his care. This is particularly relevant for Ansel's parents as they have not been able to be as successful in their employment as they would like. Because of their consistent last-minute absences, their unanticipated, yet regularly occurring, trips to pick up Ansel from school, and the frequent medical visits, Ansel's parents have had to find employment that allowed them flexibility or have had to bounce from job to job. Financial concerns have become pressing for them. Because Ansel receives services from the state, he will be eligible for housing in a supported residential program, where he will live with other adults with autism and developmental disabilities along with staff, who are present 24 hours a day. While they have not yet identified the specific housing solution, his parents anticipate interviewing the staff at the various programs in the hope of finding a setting with compassionate residential workers. Ansel's parents have also not yet solidified consistent day programming, which should involve activities to ensure that Ansel remains engaged in the community. But they are actively looking at options in the community and working with the state vocational rehabilitation program, hoping to find volunteer or employment placement so that he can engage in the community at least part-time.

While the future is unclear for Ansel, an important point is that had Ansel had the opportunities available to him as a young boy that current science has identified, such as earlier screening and diagnosis and early, intensive behavioral interventions, Ansel's life might be different now.

With gains made in science, it is entirely possible that Ansel could have been diagnosed in early toddlerhood and his intensive behavioral intervention could have started at that age, when his brain was still highly plastic and most responsive to treatment. The opportunities that exist today because of the explosion of recent scientific findings are vastly different from those offered even a decade—and certainly two decades—ago.

Each of these children and their families are unique, and their stories illustrate the many paths that autism can take. In all cases, through persistence, knowledge, and the help and support of professionals, friends, and family, the children gained skills and found their place in the world. We next describe a few takeaways from these stories.

Lessons from the Spectrum

The preceding stories illustrate the wide diversity of individuals along the autism spectrum and how recognizing their uniqueness can enable families to meet their needs optimally while protecting the well-being of the whole family. As you go forward, keep in mind the following points, which will guide you well along this path.

• *The challenges associated with ASD result from a complex interplay between biology—partly rooted in genes and partly in epigenetic effects—and environmental context.* Critically, autism is not caused by poor parenting or immunizations, nor is it caused by a single factor. Autism has many causes, which likely contributes to the incredible variability we see across children diagnosed with autism. The study of epigenetics has shown us that the environment (primarily the early uterine environment) plays a bigger role than previously thought, operating in tandem with genetic liability. This interplay is what some of the families in the stories above were able to use to their advantage. By changing some aspects of the complex mix affecting their child, they were able to help their child develop most effectively—for Milo it was behavioral intervention focused on directing his attention to the social world, while for Billy it was managing sleep hygiene, which in turn improved his ability to manage his autism symptoms.

• **What works for a child won't necessarily pay off right away.** But in each case above, once the family found the right mix, the situation began to turn around within weeks or months. While there are no guarantees, *this really does happen, and it can happen for you.*

• **Professional support and personal lifestyle changes can augment each other nicely.** For the families described above, it was important to balance the realization that a child's environment can make a real difference in her success with acceptance of the need for some professional help as well—at some point, in some way, in most cases. In fact, the combination of the two is the most common picture in successful progress for children with autism. Lifestyle changes are likely to help, and to amplify the benefit of professional help or reduce the amount of it you need, but they won't be a panacea.

• **The principles we are talking about apply whether or not a child formally meets the diagnostic criteria for autism.** Autism is probably the extreme end of a dimension spanning the full range of social abilities. Wherever a child is on that continuum, if she is being impaired by these problems, then the research summarized in this book may be relevant. If your efforts to manage the problems on your own aren't working, get a professional evaluation. Use the guidelines for what to look for in Chapter 5. Whether or not your child gets a diagnosis of autism, the evaluation can help clarify the nature of the problem, and the professional can help you fine-tune how you implement your strategy. Whether it is behavioral management, medication, or, for that matter, sleep training, the intervention can range from ineffective to very effective depending in part on how carefully it is implemented. Getting the right team in your corner can help you make sure you hit all the right notes.

• **The family dynamics described in this chapter can occur in almost any cultural context.** We have heard stories like those described above in observant Christian, Muslim, and Jewish homes as well as in secular and nonreligious homes, and in families that are white, African American, Hispanic/Latino, Asian American, and of mixed race. We work in the United States, but our colleagues in many other countries write and talk about very recognizable situations when we meet at conferences. In each of these cultural and social contexts, there are of course additional complexities to consider that make your situation unique and specific.

- *Changes to your family's routines and decisions about treatment for your child should always be based on what makes the most sense for your child, you, and your family.* Take a look at your own situation. You may be at the beginning of the journey and want to know what to do first. Or perhaps you feel like you have already tried every medication or complementary intervention to no avail. Maybe you've taken measures to improve your child's social communication through speech therapy but not addressed challenging behaviors that are impeding his ability to use those newfound social communication skills. As we mentioned earlier in this book, the best place to start is the diagnostic evaluation report you received (or if it has been a while, a comprehensive assessment report that you've recently received). Check in with those professional recommendations and think through your options—based on what you intuitively think might work best for your child but also on what you can realistically manage. Clinic-based social skills instruction may seem impractical (or simply not be available) for you, while a social skills group in your child's school could easily be woven into your lives—that's just one example among many. See where the report leads you and then always be willing to revise and try something different after giving your first choices a reasonable test period.

WORKING WITH PROFESSIONALS

In Chapter 5 we reviewed what the science tells us about the various types of professional help for children with autism and their families. We highlighted the qualifications you should seek to ensure that you will get qualified help and described the circumstances that might call for particular types of help in diagnosis and treatment. But professional treatment is, of course, a two-way street. Even when you find professionals that you like and trust, you will have to feel comfortable establishing a balance between following their recommendations and making your own questions and concerns known. The pro will appreciate it when you have done some homework, have some ideas, and are motivated. At the same time, if you aren't going to follow their advice, most professionals will wonder why you called them in the first place. So be open to the professionals' recommendations, recognizing that a good professional will also listen to your ideas. Ideally, a meeting of the minds will take place. Good clinicians will be comfortable explaining why a particular idea isn't suitable in your child's case, will understand that sometimes their first suggestion won't work, or, quite often, will help you try your own idea in a safe and supported way.

For example, when Jessica originally took Milo to his pediatrician, the pediatrician cautioned waiting and watching. During that second visit, when Jessica highlighted the additional challenges she saw in Milo beyond language delays, the pediatrician reconsidered and further explored what Jessica's concerns were. After that careful line of questioning, the doctor made a referral for Milo to have a diagnostic evaluation for autism.

As another example, Jen brought Georgia in to see a psychiatrist to try to develop an approach to help manage an increase in agitation that she and Steven were observing during transitions. The family incorporated a number of social stories and picture schedules into their routine, but given Georgia's cognitive challenges it was difficult to determine if she was understanding these approaches. The psychiatrist tried a new medication to help address some suspected anxiety that could be contributing to the agitation that accompanied transitions. They were given a prescription and told to come back in 3 months. But after one month on the prescription, they could see that, while Georgia was managing transitions better, she seemed lethargic and even less engaged with her family than usual. They did not know what to do—there was less agitation, but Jen felt like her daughter was disappearing. They returned to the psychiatrist, who speculated that the dosage simply needed adjustment. The psychiatrist agreed to check in with the family for several consecutive weeks, adjusting the dose until the balance between reduced agitation and stable engagement with the family was reached.

Questions to Ask the Professionals

Here's a short list of questions you can productively ask any clinician you're considering for diagnosis and treatment of your child. You won't necessarily ask every single question, but rather you can draw on those suggested questions that are relevant to your situation. Your goal is to be an active partner in the process and let your clinician know you want to learn and understand. These questions can help you feel comfortable with your professionals and also help both you and them avoid mistakes. A good professional will appreciate that and be glad you are so engaged. She won't run every test you suggest (nor should she, if it's not needed), but she should have a well-thought-out answer to these questions and appreciate the chance to clarify her thinking. Some of these questions may be answered in advance on the clinician's web page or other marketing materials.

Professional Background

- "What is your degree in?"
- "Are you fully licensed in this state?"
- "How long have you been doing this work?"
- "What types of cases or problems do you consider to be your strong suit?"
- "Do you specialize in children [or toddlers or teenagers or adults]?"
- "Do you specialize in autism?"
- "What do you need from me to enable you to be maximally helpful to me?"

Diagnostics

- "Are you confident these challenges are not better explained by intellectual impairment/cognitive abilities?"
- "He has a lot of tantrums, and he also has problems getting organized. I've heard these can be connected. Is it possible this is all related to ADHD and not autism?"
- "She seems compelled to do certain routines repetitively. It seems to be compulsive. How do you know this is autism and not anxiety?"
- "He has limited interest in others, and his irritability seems

unrelated to events that I can figure out. How do we know it's not depression?"

- "What are the reasons you think this is autism? What should I be watching for that would indicate we need a fresh review of diagnostics?"
- "What else can I watch for or should I be looking out for?"

Treatments

- "What will be the most effective interventions for *my* child?"
- "Are the treatments you are recommending based on evidence?"
- "What are things that I could be doing at home to help interventions my child is getting [at school, clinic, etc.]?"
- "What treatments and interventions should I start first?"
- "Can you help me establish a bedtime routine (or morning routine to get out the door)?"
- "What challenges is this medication targeting for my child?"
- "How are you selecting which medication to try?"
- "Is this dose a high dose, low dose, or medium dose?"
- "Why don't we try a different dose of the medication before we change medicines?"
- "Some things are going better now, but some things have gotten worse. Can we modify our approach?"
- "Can I have a list of side effects to watch for?"
- "Do you provide parent behavioral counseling? What does that consist of?"
- "Do you follow a certain model or curriculum when you teach parenting skills?"
- "How many meetings will we plan on?"
- "How will we evaluate our progress?"

Self-Care

- "I've been preoccupied by my own problems/mood/conflicts in marriage or at work/health problems/other. Do you think addressing that would help my child? Do you think it is feasible? Can you give me an appropriate referral?"

WHAT'S AHEAD FOR YOUR CHILD?

Perhaps the most pressing concern for parents who have a child with autism or a similar developmental issue is "What does the future hold?" We don't have a crystal ball. If we did, joining the circus and traveling the world telling fortunes might prove to be a more helpful career than academic medicine. But in the absence of the crystal ball all we can do is look to our experience and see what the science shows. We have seen firsthand what the research shows in the thousands of children with autism we've worked with, in the many families we've partnered with in research studies, and in the families we've communicated with at talks, community events, and meetings—that many children with ASD reach a positive outcome. Throughout the book we've mentioned several resilience factors for children and those transitioning into adulthood, but in the end, we circle back to the big-picture priorities for you as a parent. The nonnegotiables are the same whether your child is thriving or struggling. The children who do well invariably had parents who were able to do the following:

1. *Developed strong advocacy skills for their children.* They showed the community what their child needed, and they made sure their child got that. Sometimes they did so smoothly and easily and other times the advocacy involved the legal system and lots of tears and hurt feelings. Ultimately they recognized what their child needed, learned how to get that, and made sure their child got it.

2. *Stayed engaged with their kids—through thick and thin.* They never disconnected, gave up, or lost interest. These children knew that no matter what else anybody might say, and no matter how many mistakes they might make, their parents were in it with them for the long haul.

3. *Were aware that their own mental and physical health were important and took care of themselves.* These parents tried to work out their own depression, alcohol abuse, past trauma, stress, and marital conflicts by reading self-help books, seeing a counselor, talking to friends, or engaging in

self-examination. As a result, even while they may have felt they were making the same mistakes year after year, they were aware of their own actions, able to hear the perspective of their children, and able to adapt when possible.

4. *Assembled a team.* These parents knew that "it takes a village." They found others who were also strong advocates for their children, who kept their child's best interests in the foreground, which ensured that the parents were not alone in their efforts to provide the best support for their child.

5. *Became an autism expert.* That doesn't mean the parents all went to medical school or earned a graduate degree specializing in autism intervention. But these parents educated themselves on what the science says, asked questions of their child's providers, familiarized themselves with their community resources, and made sure they knew what autism was like for their child. In this way they made sure that their child was going to get the best support possible. We are proud to say that by reading this book you are already tackling this item directly!

6. *Formed a strong social support network.* They relied on other parents, friends, and family for emotional, social, and logistical support. They weren't afraid to ask for help when they needed it. They developed friendships with supportive people who cared about them and with whom they could share both their struggles and their victories. They found time for fun and laughter with their support group.

When we say the children are doing well, we don't mean that all of them ended up in a regular education classroom or moved to New York City to perform on Broadway or whatever other hope that parents have shared with us over the years. But we mean that the kids and families achieved goals and outcomes that worked for them. For Georgia's family the goal was that their family be together every day for dinner and participate in community activities as a family. For Ansel and his family, the goal was to have Ansel stay in school until he was 21 and then live outside the home and engage in meaningful activity. For Jessica, who shared this comment using her favorite tactic of humor, her goal for Milo was that he would stop licking the neighbor's doorstep. These families were able to achieve their goals because the parents exhibited the resilience factors listed above.

And what if you feel like you fall short on some of them? That doesn't mean you can't also get your kids to a positive outcome. We just want to emphasize that hitting these targets markedly raises the odds.

We can't overemphasize the importance of self-care. Stress may be perhaps the most underappreciated influence on child outcomes. When a parent is overly stressed, it's very difficult to provide the necessary support and implement the interventions needed. Furthermore, caring for a child with autism is hard. It's challenging, draining, demanding, and exhausting. Without an occasional break, without getting your own exercise and sleep, having a supportive friend or peer group for yourself, and some good times in your own life, it is very difficult to sustain the journey you need to take with your child. Take care of yourself, and take care of your child. Many of the changes in lifestyle discussed here will help you as well as your child and can be done together as a family.

WHERE IS THE SCIENCE HEADED?

In the field of psychology, we say that the best predictor of future behavior is past behavior. So what happens when we apply that concept here? When we look at past "scientific behavior," we see massive growth in our understanding of the causes of autism and how we can best support individuals with autism, with scientists and families working together.

A little over 10 years ago we knew relatively little about the causes of autism compared to today, and the outlook for those with autism was too often seen as hopeless. As we discussed in the first chapters of this book, understanding the causes is critical because it can allow us to figure out ways to most effectively support individuals and their families. In the past decade we have seen remarkable progress on several fronts. On the genetic front, public and private investment increased dramatically and spurred partnerships that enabled the identification of several specific rare genes with major effects, providing hope for an understanding of biological pathways. First, the identification of genes and genetic events highlighted the possibility that genetic contributions interact through complex patterns with the early environment. For the first time we had a biological understanding of the adage "If you've met one individual with autism . . . you've met one individual with autism." Second, the identification of these genes, along with dramatic progress in brain-imaging technology and an explosion of brain-imaging studies, helped illuminate the way that brain structures develop and function in autism, as we discussed in Chapter 4.

Progress on clinical studies clarified that ASD is better seen as a spectrum—this broadening and unifying of the spectrum was critical to the genetic progress we just mentioned and exemplifies the important synergy between progress in clinical description and progress in research on causes and mechanisms—one cannot progress without the other. On the basic science side, a wealth of understanding has emerged around epigenetic mechanisms and the way in which environments can get under the skin and shape biology—and help us identify potentially reversible causes.

The combination of these lines of progress has in turn started to pave the way for the development of targeted supports for individuals with autism and novel ways to monitor treatment effectiveness. Indeed, in the past decade progress in treatment studies and early detection has opened up new hope that children with ASD may recover far more often and more fully than was previously thought possible.

So, using that "past behavior" to predict "future behavior," we can anticipate more progress on multiple lines at once—on clinical description and early identification, on identifying reversible environmental inputs and how they work biologically to affect brain development, and on understanding what genes are doing in the brain in ways that may lead to new treatment ideas and better diagnostics. We are sure to see further exciting, large-scale collaborative efforts by scientists across the globe working together with families to focus on issues that are critical to the field; but we will also see individual laboratories striking out in novel directions and opening up new ideas. All of this will help move us further toward answering the core question: How do we best help support individuals with autism to become the people they want to be? This research will include work toward earlier detection, advances in precision medicine, and the identification of biological markers for treatment monitoring, as well as efforts to educate the general public on the importance of inclusion and integration with the community, particularly as children transition into adulthood.

Neurodevelopmental disorders like ASD and ADHD, mental

disorders like depression, anxiety, and schizophrenia, and addictive disorders are collectively the world's number-one cause of morbidity compared to any other disease category ("morbidity" is defined formally as years lived with disease or disability, but for our purposes it means a cumulative loss of quality of life over the lifetime). This is because these disorders emerge in childhood, during the long period of brain development, and they are chronic. Although public and private investment in autism research has increased impressively in the past decade, we still don't fund enough research on autism or on neurodevelopmental conditions generally relative to their social cost. As a society, we do a better job funding research on what kills us when we are old after a full life than on conditions that can rob kids of their future when they are young. That may change, and we believe it will, because progress to date is impressive and exciting. The energy in the scientific community is high, and the future is bright for new treatments and discoveries.

There is ample reason for optimism and hope in your own life too. Autism is considered a lifelong disorder, but we know now that, with the right supports, every person with autism can learn new skills and lead a meaningful life. Through better public awareness, employers and society at large are not only becoming more informed about and accepting of autism, but have also come to appreciate the unique strengths and perspectives that people on the spectrum bring to the world. Science shows that children and adults on the autism spectrum continue to improve their skills throughout life. We now understand more about the challenges associated with ASD and how to address them. More than ever, the future is hopeful for individuals with ASD and their families. Our hope is that this book will provide meaningful advice along the way and that it will help your child reach his or her full potential.

RESOURCES

GENERAL INFORMATION REGARDING ASD

National Library of Medicine: Autism
The National Library of Medicine compiles comprehensive information and fact sheets about ASD.
www.nlm.nih.gov/medlineplus/autism.html

Spectrum: Autism Research News
Spectrum provides easily digestible, comprehensive news and analysis about autism research.
www.spectrumnews.org

International Society for Autism Research (INSAR)
INSAR maintains a website reporting on activities of this organization focused on promoting autism research.
www.autism-insar.org/default.aspx

Centers for Disease Control and Prevention (CDC)
The CDC has an authoritative site dedicated to ASD.
www.cdc.gov/ncbddd/autism

National Institute of Mental Health (NIMH)
The NIMH provides an authoritative summary of facts about ASD.
www.nimh.nih.gov/health/topics/autism-spectrum-disorders-asd/index.shtml

INFORMATION FOR PARENTS, FAMILIES, AND INDIVIDUALS IMPACTED BY ASD

American Academy of Pediatrics (AAP)
The AAP is an excellent source of information about all aspects of children's health, including ASD.
www.aap.org

The Arc
The Arc's mission is to promote and protect the human rights of people with intellectual and developmental disabilities. There are chapters throughout each state.
www.thearc.org

Autistica
Autistica is a UK-based charity organization that supports autism research.
www.autistica.org.uk/about-us/about-us

Autism Science Foundation (ASF)
The ASF is a U.S.-based autism research support organization.
https://autismsciencefoundation.org

Autism Society
The Autism Society has information available in both English and Spanish and maintains general information about autism.
www.autism-society.org
Spanish: *www.autism-society.org/site/PageServer?pagename=autismo*

Autism Speaks
Autism Speaks maintains a large variety of information and many resources and downloadable tools for parents and individuals impacted by ASD.
www.autismspeaks.org

Canadian Paediatric Society (CPS)
The CPS serves both CPS members and other health care professionals with information they need to make informed decisions about child health care.
www.cps.ca

First Signs
The First Signs organization maintains information about monitoring childhood development, the screening and referral process, and support for concerns. One of the tools is the ASD Video Glossary.
http://firstsigns.org

National Autistic Society
The National Autistic Society, based in the United Kingdom, offers a
wide range of support services for people with autism, including diagnosis
information, skills training, social and educational programs, access support,
and advocacy.
www.autism.org.uk

Psychiatric Times
Psychiatric Times is a monthly online publication offering feature articles,
clinical news, and reports on special topics from expert writers across a broad
range of psychiatric issues involving children and adults.
www.psychiatrictimes.com

Raising Children Network
This is a comprehensive website for Australian parents, offering resources,
discussion forums, videos, and more, including information on autism.
Articles have age keys so parents and kids can read them.
http://raisingchildren.net.au

SCIENCE RESOURCES SPECIFICALLY REGARDING NEUROSCIENCE, GENETICS, AND EPIGENETICS

The American Society for Human Genetics (ASHG) has a basic primer on
genetics.
www.ashg.org/education/everyone_1.shtml

Brain Connection, sponsored by BrainHQ, a group promoting cognitive brain
training, provides a variety of articles and resources about brain development
and new brain research, including several articles on children's learning.
https://brainconnection.brainhq.com

The Society for Neuroscience website provides a rich, accessible set of
information modules for the general public.
www.brainfacts.org

The Guardian has put together a well-written lay summary of the key points of
epigenetics.
*www.theguardian.com/science/occams-corner/2014/apr/25/epigenetics-beginners-guide-
to-everything*

The National Institutes of Health (NIH) has a website for its epigenetics
consortium that occasionally posts cutting-edge plans and breakthroughs
(http://ihec-epigenomes.org) that also include videos and tutorials

(http://ihec-epigenomes.org/why-epigenomics/video-clips), as well as links to other resources under its "About" and "Why Epigenomics" links.

There is a nice article in *The New Yorker* by Siddhartha Mukherjee regarding epigenetics.
www.newyorker.com/magazine/2016/05/02/breakthroughs-in-epigenetics

The subscription magazine *Scientific American* covers new developments in cognitive neuroscience accessible to the layperson.
www.scientificamerican.com/mind

The journal *Nature*'s resource library, called Scitable, has a summary of key information regarding epigenetics.
www.nature.com/scitable/topicpage/epigenetic-influences-and-disease-895

IDENTIFICATION, DIAGNOSIS, AND TREATMENT RESOURCES

Autism Speaks Resource Guide
The resource guide is an online database for clinical and support resources searchable by where you live, life stage, and level of support needed.
www.autismspeaks.org/resource-guide

Autism Speaks First Concern to Action Kit
This kit provides guidance for what to do if you have concerns about autism in your young child.
www.autismspeaks.org/tool-kit/first-concern-action-tool-kit

Autism Speaks 100 Day Kit
The Autism Speaks 100 Day Kit contains freely available information for families whose children have recently been diagnosed with ASD to help prioritize the most essential steps in the 100 days following the diagnosis.
www.autismspeaks.org/tool-kit/100-day-kit-young-children
www.autismspeaks.org/tool-kit/100-day-kit-school-age-children

Autism Screening, Diagnosis, and Treatment Guidelines
The CDC website provides guidelines issued by the American Academy of Pediatrics, American Academy of Neurology, and Child Neurology Society.
www.cdc.gov/ncbddd/autism/hcp-recommendations.html

Interactive Tools to Track Child Development from the CDC
The CDC offers interactive tools to help parents track how a child plays, learns, speaks, and acts. Interactive Milestone Charts and a checklist are offered that teach parents about developmental milestones to help them recognize when development may be off course. They also offer a video called

Baby Steps: Learn the Signs. Act Early, which provides information and guidance on identifying developmental disabilities.
www.cdc.gov/ncbddd/actearly/milestones

National Autism Center's National Standards Project
The National Autism Center's National Standards Project offers evidence-based information about the effectiveness of interventions for individuals with ASD.
www.nationalautismcenter.org/national-standards-project

National Center for Complementary and Integrative Health (NCCIH)
The NCCIH, an agency of the NIH, provides a comprehensive overview of complementary and alternative medicines and treatments.
https://nccih.nih.gov

SELECT ACADEMIC CLINICAL RESEARCH CENTERS

Center for Autism and the Developing Brain, White Plains, NY
www.nyp.org/psychiatry/services/center-for-autism-and-the-developing-brain

Duke Center for Autism and Brain Development, Durham, NC
https://autismcenter.duke.edu

Marcus Autism Center, Atlanta, GA
www.marcus.org

Nationwide Children's Center for ASD, Columbus, OH
www.nationwidechildrens.org/specialties/center-for-autism-spectrum-disorders

Seattle Children's Autism Center, Seattle, WA
www.seattlechildrens.org/clinics/autism-center

Seaver Center at Mt. Sinai Medical Center, New York, NY
https://icahn.mssm.edu/research/seaver

TEACCH Autism Program, Chapel Hill, NC
https://teacch.com

UC Davis MIND Institute, Davis, CA
https://health.ucdavis.edu/mindinstitute

UCLA Center for Autism Research and Treatment, Los Angeles, CA
www.semel.ucla.edu/autism

STAR Center for Autism and Neurodevelopmental Disorders,
San Francisco, CA
https://star.ucsf.edu

UW Autism Center, Seattle, WA
https://depts.washington.edu/uwautism

NUTRITION AND DIET

Food Allergy Research and Education (FARE)
Parents and educators can find detailed suggestions and information about
food allergies at this CDC-sponsored site.
www.foodallergy.org

Guidelines and tips for healthy nutritional planning for your child are
available at the National Institutes of Health *(https://medlineplus.gov/
childnutrition.html)* and the USDA *(http://fnic.nal.usda.gov/lifecycle-nutrition/child-
nutrition)*.

SLEEP

The National Sleep Foundation website provides background information,
checklists, and guidelines.
https://sleepfoundation.org

Sleep behavior programs are outlined at *http://drcraigcanapari.com/at-long-last-
sleep-training-tools-for-the-exhausted-parent*.

EXERCISE

The CDC provides clear exercise guidelines, lists of moderate activities for
different ages, and suggestions on getting activity into your child's life.
www.cdc.gov/physicalactivity/basics/children/index.htm.

The CDC's Body and Mind (BAM!) website has interactive tools for you
and your child and information on how to participate in dozens of different
individual and group activities, games, and sports to help you identify suitable
activities.
www.cdc.gov/bam/activity/index.html

The University of Texas CATCH (Coordinated Approach to Child Health)
curriculum for schools and educators, designed to prevent childhood obesity,

offers programs aimed at increasing moderate to vigorous exercise, including a family/home module.
http://catchinfo.org/about

TECHNOLOGY

The Common Sense Media website provides information, advice, and tools to help sift through media options (movies, games, etc.) to make informed decisions.
www.commonsensemedia.org

Children's Technology Review provides professional reviews of interactive technology (software, video games) to aid in monitoring and choosing products to use.
www.childrenssoftware.com

TRANSITION PLANNING

Autism Speaks Transition Kit
www.autismspeaks.org/tool-kit/transition-tool-kit

The Columbia Regional Program Transition Toolkit provides transition team members with practical information and easy access to resources to aid in the transition process.
www.crporegon.org/Page/175

IRISS, a social service agency based in Scotland, provides a nice summary of information regarding transition.
www.iriss.org.uk/sites/default/files/iriss-insight-5.pdf

STRESS REDUCTION

The American Psychological Association has a comprehensive page outlining the impact of stress on the body and helpful tips on stress management.
www.apa.org/helpcenter/stress/index

The CDC has a good summary of basic strategies to help you and your kids prevent or handle too much stress.
www.cdc.gov/violenceprevention/pub/coping_with_stress_tips.html

Medline Plus, offered by the U.S. National Library of Medicine, has a nice resource regarding psychological stress with information, tips, resources, and links.
https://medlineplus.gov/stress.html

The University of Nebraska Medical Center has a good list of relaxation apps that are freely available for download.
www.unmc.edu/wellness/_documents/FreeRelaxApps.pdf

The U.S. Department of Health and Human Services website provides information regarding stress management approaches.
https://healthfinder.gov/HealthTopics/Category/health-conditions-and-diseases/heart-health/manage-stress

WebMD's MedicineNet shares information regarding stress and stress management.
www.medicinenet.com/stress/article.htm

PERSON-CENTERED PLANNING

The Arc provides information regarding person-centered planning.
https://arcofkingcounty.org/resource-guide/personcentered-planning/person-centered-planning.html

Informing Families is a Washington State Developmental Disabilities Council resource that provides information regarding person-centered planning.
http://informingfamilies.org/pcp

SEX EDUCATION

The National Autistic Society (U.K.) has good information and tips for families regarding sexual education.
www.autism.org.uk/sexeducation

Planned Parenthood has a good article on sex education for children and teens with autism.
www.plannedparenthood.org/planned-parenthood-massachusetts/local-training-education/parent-buzz-newsletter/parent-buzz-e-newsletters/sexuality-education-youth-autism-spectrum

VeryWellHealth.Com has a brief article on sex education for teens with autism.
www.verywellhealth.com/autism-sex-education-260490

ADVOCACY

Arc chapters in every state provide opportunities to learn about advocacy for people with intellectual and developmental disabilities.
www.thearc.org

Autism Speaks Advocacy Kit
www.autismspeaks.org/tool-kit/advocacy-tool-kit

HOUSING RESOURCES

Autism Housing Network
This program provides information, resources, and tools focused on housing.
www.autismhousingnetwork.org

Autism Speaks Housing Kit
www.autismspeaks.org/tool-kit/housing-and-residential-supports-tool-kit

Autism After 16
The article "Gimme Shelter: Housing for Adults with Autism" appears in the
online newsletter *Autism After 16*.
www.autismafter16.com/article/10-19-2011/gimme-shelter-housing-adults-autism

The HUD website provides a fact sheet on Section 8 vouchers and housing.
www.hud.gov/topics/housing_choice_voucher_program_section_8

Use this web page to find HUD information for your state.
http://portal.hud.gov/hudportal/HUD?src=/states/washington/offices

EMPLOYMENT

Autism Speaks Employment Kit
www.autismspeaks.org/tool-kit/employment-tool-kit

Choose Work
The U.S. Social Security Administration (SSA) provides employment support
services for individuals receiving Social Security disability benefits. (You can
use the SSA website, listed below under Financial Resources, to apply for
benefits.)
https://choosework.ssa.gov

Hire Autism
Hire Autism is a program of the Organization for Autism Research focused on
job placement for individuals with autism.
https://hireautism.org

Uptimize and Autism Research Institute Job Training Video for individuals
with autism
http://uptimize.com/on-demand-training

FINANCIAL RESOURCES

ABLE accounts
Information regarding ABLE accounts is located online.
www.ablenrc.org

Autism Speaks Financial Planning Kit
www.autismspeaks.org/tool-kit/financial-planning-tool-kit

Medicaid
This web page ("Autism Services") describes and provides links to government
publications that offer guidance on Medicaid benefits for individuals with
autism.
www.medicaid.gov/medicaid/benefits/autism/index.html

**National Association of State Directors of Developmental Disabilities
Services (NASDDDS)**
This organization's website provides contact information for all of the
state agencies supporting individuals with intellectual and developmental
disabilities (the names vary by state).
www.nasddds.org/state-agencies

U.S. Social Security Administration (SSA)
The SSA provides funding resources via two channels: Supplemental Security
Income (SSI) and Social Security disability insurance.
www.socialsecurity.gov

EDUCATION RESOURCES

Autism Speaks IEP Kit
*www.autismspeaks.org/tool-kit/individualized-education-program-iep-summary-
process-and-practical-tips*

Autism Speaks Postsecondary Education Kit
www.autismspeaks.org/tool-kit/postsecondary-educational-opportunities-guide

Office of Special Education Programs
The U.S. Department of Education provides a transition guide for schools and
educators to use for planning postsecondary education and employment.
https://sites.ed.gov/idea/files/postsecondary-transition-guide-may-2017.pdf

Think College
Think College is a resource with programs designed to expand postsecondary education opportunities for individuals with disabilities.
https://thinkcollege.net

Wrightslaw
The Wrightslaw website provides information related to special education law, the development of IEPs, and advocacy for children with disabilities.
www.wrightslaw.com

LEGAL RESOURCES

Administration for Community Living
This organization provides information about state protection and advocacy programs along with links to each state's programs.
https://acl.gov/programs/aging-and-disability-networks/state-protection-advocacy-systems

Autism Speaks
Autism Speaks offers legal information on its website.
www.autismspeaks.org/your-childs-rights

Autism Society
A summary of legal information is provided on this organization's website.
www.autism-society.org/living-with-autism/legal-resources

VeryWellHealth.Com
You can find legal and advocacy information and guidance for families at this link.
www.verywellhealth.com/guardianship-for-adults-with-autism-4165687

REFERENCES

The following are the key sources for the studies mentioned and research findings discussed in the text.

CHAPTER 1: A NEW UNDERSTANDING OF AUTISM SPECTRUM DISORDER

American Psychiatric Association. (1986). *Diagnostic and statistical manual of mental disorders* (DSM-III-R) (3rd ed., rev.). Washington, DC: Author.

American Psychiatric Association. (1994). *Diagnostic and statistical manual of mental disorders* (DSM-IV) (4th ed.). Washington, DC: Author

American Psychiatric Association. (2013). *Diagnostic and statistical manual of mental disorders* (DSM-5) (5th ed.). Arlington, VA: Author.

Arnett, A., Trinh, S., & Bernier, R. (2018). The state of research on the genetics of autism spectrum disorder: Methodological, clinical and conceptual progress. *Current Opinion in Psychology, 27,* 1–5.

Barger, B., Campbell, J., & McDonough, J. (2013). Prevalence and onset of regression within autism spectrum disorders: A meta-analytic review. *Journal of Autism and Developmental Disorders, 43*(4), 817–828.

Bernier, R. (2012, March 20). How do we measure autism severity? *SFARI Viewpoint.*

Bernier, R., & Dawson, G. (2016). Autism spectrum disorders. In D. Cicchetti (Ed.), *Developmental psychopathology* (Vol. 3, 3rd ed.). New York: Wiley.

Constantino, J. N., & Charman, T. (2012). Gender bias, female resilience, and the sex ratio in autism. *Journal of the American Academy of Child and Adolescent Psychiatry, 51*(8), 756–758.

Dawson, G., & Bernier, R. (2013). A quarter century of progress in the detection and early treatment of autism spectrum disorder. *Development and Psychopathology, 25,* 1455–1472.

Dawson, G., Bernier, R., & Ring, R. (2012). Social attention: A possible early response indicator in autism clinical trials. *Journal of Neurodevelopmental Disorders, 4,* 11–35.

Fein, D., Barton, M., & Dumont-Mathieu, T. (2017). Optimizing outcome in autism spectrum disorders. *Policy Insights from the Behavioral and Brain Sciences, 4*(1), 71–78.

Fein, D., Barton, M., Eigsti, I.-M., Kelley, E., Naigles, L., Schultz, R. T., et al. (2013).

Optimal outcome in individuals with a history of autism. *Journal of Child Psychology and Psychiatry, 54,* 195–205.

Folstein, S., & Rutter, M. (1977). Infantile autism: A genetic study of 21 twin pairs. *Journal of Child Psychology and Psychiatry,18*(4), 297–321.

Georgiades, S., & Kasari, C. (2018). Reframing optimal outcomes in autism. *JAMA Pediatrics, 172*(8), 716–717.

Informed Health Online. (2016, June 15). *What types of studies are there?* Cologne, Germany: Institute for Quality and Efficiency in Health Care. Retrieved from *www. ncbi.nlm.nih.gov/books/NBK390304.*

Jacquemont, S., Coe, B. P., Hersch, M., Duyzend, M. H., Krumm, N., Bergmann, S., et al. (2014). A higher mutational burden in females supports a "female protective model" in neurodevelopmental disorders. *American Journal of Human Genetics, 94*(3), 415–425.

Jones, W., & Klin, A. (2013). Attention to eyes is present but in decline in 2- to 6-month-old infants later diagnosed with autism. *Nature, 504*(7480), 427–431.

Kanner, L. (1943). Autistic disturbances of affective contact. *Nervous Child, 2,* 217–250.

King, B., Navot, N., Bernier, R., & Webb, S. (2014). Update on diagnostic classification in autism. *Current Opinion in Psychiatry, 27,* 105–109.

Krumm, N., Turner, T., Baker, C., Vives, L, Mohajeri, K., Witherspoon, K., et al. (2015). Excess of rare, inherited truncating mutations in autism. *Nature Genetics, 47*(6), 582–588.

Kurita, H. (1985). Infantile autism with speech loss before the age of thirty months. *Journal of the American Academy of Child Psychiatry 24*(2), 191–196.

Lai, M. C., Lombardo, M. V., Auyeung, B., Chakrabarti, B., & Baron-Cohen, S. (2015). Sex/gender differences and autism: Setting the scene for future research. *Journal of the American Academy of Child and Adolescent Psychiatry, 54*(1), 11–24.

Lai, M., Lombardo, M., Suckling, J., Ruigrok, A., Chakrabarti, B., Ecker, C., et al. (2013). Biological sex affects the neurobiology of autism. *Brain, 136*(9), 2799–2815.

Lord, C., Petkova, E., Hus, V., Gan, W., Martin, D. M., Ousley, O., et al. (2011). A multi-site study of the clinical diagnosis of different autism spectrum disorders. *Archives of General Psychiatry, 69*(3), 306–313.

Luyster, R., Richler, J., Risi, S., Hsu, W., Dawson, G., Bernier, R., et al. (2005). Early regression in social communication in autistic spectrum disorders: A CPEA study. *Developmental Neuropsychology, 27,* 311–336.

Mottron, L., Duret, P., Mueller, S., Moore, R., Forgeot D'Arc, B., Jacquemont, S., et al. (2015). Sex differences in brain plasticity: A new hypothesis for sex ratio bias in autism. *Molecular Autism, 6,* 33.

Nigg, J. T. (2017). *Getting ahead of ADHD: What next-generation science says about treatments that work—and how you can make them work for your child.* New York: Guilford Press.

Osterling, J., & Dawson, G. (1994). Early recognition of children with autism: A study of first birthday home videotapes. *Journal of Autism and Developmental Disorders 24*(3), 247–257.

Osterling, J., Dawson, G., & Munson, J. (2002). Early recognition of 1-year-old infants with autism spectrum disorder versus mental retardation. *Development and Psychopathology, 14*(2), 239–251.

Pearson, N., Charman, T., Happé, F., Bolton, P. F., & McEwen, F. S. (2018). Regression in autism spectrum disorder: Reconciling findings from retrospective and prospective research. *Autism Research, 11*(12), 1602–1620.

Schaer, M., Kochalka, J., Padmanabhan, A., Supekar, K., & Menon, V. (2015). Sex differences in cortical volume and gyrification in autism. *Molecular Autism, 6.*

Werner, E., & Dawson, G. (2005). Validation of the phenomenon of autistic regression using home videotapes. *Archives of General Psychiatry 62*(8), 889–895.

Wing, L., & Gould, J. (1979). Severe impairments of social interaction and associated abnormalities in children: Epidemiology and classification. *Journal of Autism Development Disorders, 9,* 11–29.

CHAPTER 2: WHAT ARE THE ESSENTIAL FEATURES THAT DEFINE THE AUTISM SPECTRUM?

Amaral, D., Dawson, G., & Geschwind, D. (2011). *Autism spectrum disorders.* New York: Oxford University Press.

Bacon, A., Fein, D., Morris, R., Waterhouse, L., & Allen, D. (1998). The responses of autistic children to the distress of others. *Journal of Autism and Developmental Disorders, 28,* 129–142.

Baron-Cohen, S. (1995). *Mindblindness: An essay on autism and theory of mind.* Cambridge, MA: Bradford/MIT Press.

Baron-Cohen, S., Baldwin, D., & Crowson, M. (1997). Do children with autism use the speaker's direction of gaze strategy to crack the code of language? *Child Development, 68,* 48–57.

Baron-Cohen, S., Leslie, A. M., & Frith, U. (1985). Does the autistic child have a theory of mind? *Cognition, 21,* 37–46.

Baron-Cohen, S., Ring, H., Bullmore, E., Wheelwright, S., Ashwin, C., & Williams, S. (2000). The amygdala theory of autism. *Neuroscience and Biobehavioral Reviews, 24,* 355–364.

Bernier, R., Dawson, G., & Webb, S. (2005). Understanding impairments in social engagement in autism. In P. Marshall & N. Fox (Eds.), *The development of social engagement: Neurobiological perspectives.* New York: Oxford University Press.

Björnsdotter, M., Wang, N., Pelphrey, K., & Kaiser, M. D. (2016). Evaluation of quantified social perception circuit activity as a neurobiological marker of autism spectrum disorder. *JAMA Psychiatry, 73*(6), 614–621.

Bodfish, J. (2011). Repetitive behaviors in individuals with autism. In D. Amaral, G. Dawson, & D. Geschwind (Eds.), *Autism spectrum disorders.* New York: Oxford University Press.

Bottema-Beutel, K., Kim, S. Y., & Crowley, S. (2019). A systematic review and meta-regression analysis of social functioning correlates in autism and typical development. *Autism Research, 12*(2), 152–175.

Chevallier, C., Kohls, G., Troiani, V., Brodkin, E., & Schultz, R. (2012). The social motivation theory of autism. *Trends in Cognitive Sciences, 16*(4), 231–239.

Dawson, G., Meltzoff, A., Osterling, J., Rinaldi, J., & Brown, E. (1998). Children with autism fail to orient to naturally occurring social stimuli. *Journal of Autism and Developmental Disorders, 28,* 479–485.

Dawson, G., Toth, K., Abbott, R., Osterling, J., Munson, J., Estes, A., et al. (2004).

Early social attention impairments in autism: Social orienting, joint attention, and attention to distress. *Developmental Psychology, 40*(2), 271–283.

Dawson, G., Webb, S. J., & McPartland, J. (2005). Understanding the nature of face processing impairment in autism: Insights from behavioral and electrophysiological studies. *Developmental Neuropsychology, 27,* 403–424.

Dichter, G., Felder, J., Green, S., Rittenberg, A., Sasson, N., & Bodfish, J. (2010). Reward circuitry function in autism spectrum disorders. *Social, Cognitive and Affective Neuroscience, 7*(2), 160–172.

Dowd, A. C., Martinez, K., Davidson, B. C., Hixon, J. G., & Neal-Beevers, A. R. (2018). Response to distress varies by social impairment and familiarity in infants at risk for autism. *Journal of Autism and Developmental Disorders, 48*(11), 3885–3898.

Frazier, T. W., Strauss, M., Klingemier, E. W., Zetzer, E. E., Hardan, A. Y., Eng, C., et al. (2017). A meta-analysis of gaze differences to social and nonsocial information between individuals with and without autism. *Journal of the American Academy of Child and Adolescent Psychiatry, 56*(7), 546–555.

Kasari, C., Sigman, M., Mundy, P., & Yirmiya, N. (1990). Affective sharing in the context of joint attention interactions of normal, autistic, and mentally retarded children. *Journal of Autism and Developmental Disorders, 20,* 87–100.

Klin, A., Jones, W., Schultz, R., Volkmar, F., & Cohen, D. (2002). Visual fixation patterns during viewing of naturalistic social situations as predictors of social competence in individuals with autism. *Archives of General Psychiatry, 59*(9), 809–816.

Klin, A., Lin, D. J., Gorrindo, P., Ramsay, G., & Jones, W. (2009). Two-year-olds with autism orient to non-social contingencies rather than biological motion. *Nature, 459,* 257–261.

Lord, C., Elsabbagh, M., Baird, G., & Veenstra-Vanderweele, J. (2018). Autism spectrum disorder. *Lancet, 392*(10146), 508–520.

Malott, R., & Shane, J. (2016). *Principles of behavior* (7th ed.). New York: Routledge.

Mason, R. A., & Just, M. A. (2009). The role of the theory-of-mind cortical network in the comprehension of narratives. *Language and Linguistics Compass, 3,* 157–174.

McPartland, J., Dawson, G., Webb, S. J., Panagiotides, H., & Carver, L. J. (2004). Event-related brain potentials reveal anomalies in temporal processing of faces in autism spectrum disorder. *Journal of Child Psychology and Psychiatry, 45,* 1235–1245.

Orefice, L. L., Zimmerman, A. L., Chirila, A. M., Sleboda, S. J., Head, J. P., & Ginty, D. D. (2016). Peripheral mechanosensory neuron dysfunction underlies tactile and behavioral deficits in mouse models of ASDs. *Cell, 166*(2), 299–313.

Pavâl, D. (2017). A dopamine hypothesis of autism spectrum disorder. *Developmental Neuroscience, 39*(5), 355–360.

Pelphrey, K., & Carter, E. (2008). Charting the typical and atypical development of the social brain. *Developmental Psychopathology, 20*(4), 1081–1102.

Robertson, C. E., & Baron-Cohen, S. (2017). Sensory perception in autism. *Nature Reviews Neuroscience, 18*(11), 671.

Saxe, R., & Kanwisher, N. (2003). People thinking about thinking people: The role of the temporo-parietal junction in "theory of mind." *NeuroImage, 19,* 1835–1842.

Scott-Van Zeeland, A. A., Dapretto, M., Ghahremani, D. G., Poldrack, R. A., & Bookheimer, S. Y. (2010). Reward processing in autism. *Autism Research, 3,* 53–67.

Sulzer-Azaroff, B., & Mayer, R. (1991). *Behavior analysis for lasting change.* Fort Worth, TX: Holt, Reinhart & Winston.

Szatmari, P., Chawarska, K., Dawson, G., Georgiades, S., Landa, R., Lord, C., et al. (2016). Prospective longitudinal studies of infant siblings of children with autism: Lessons learned and future directions. *Journal of the American Academy of Child and Adolescent Psychiatry, 55*(3), 179–187.

Vismara, L. A., & Rogers, S. J. (2010). Behavioral treatments in autism spectrum disorder: What do we know? *Annual Review of Clinical Psychology, 27,* 447–468.

Weigelt, S., Koldewyn, K., & Kanwisher, N. (2012). Face identity recognition in autism spectrum disorders: A review of behavioral studies. *Neuroscience and Biobehavioral Reviews, 36*(3), 1060–1084.

Weiss, J., Thomson, K., & Chan, L. (2014). A systematic literature review of emotion regulation measurement in individuals with autism spectrum disorder. *Autism Research, 7*(6), 629–648.

Will, E., & Hepburn, S. (2015). Applied behavior analysis for children with neurogenetic disorders. In R. Hodapp & D. Fidler (Eds.), *International Review of Research in Developmental Disabilities* (Vol. 49, pp. 229–259). Waltham, MA: Academic Press.

Williams, D. L., Siegel, M., Mazefsky, C. A., & Autism and Developmental Disorders Inpatient Research Collaborative (2017). Problem behaviors in autism spectrum disorder: Association with verbal ability and adapting/coping skills. *Journal of Autism and Developmental Disorders, 48*(11), 1–10.

Wimmer, H., & Perner, J. (1983). Beliefs about beliefs: Representation and constraining function of wrong beliefs in young children's understanding of deception. *Cognition, 13,* 103–128.

Zhang, J., Meng, Y., He, J., Xiang, Y., Wu, C., Wang, S., et al. (2019). McGurk Effect by individuals with autism spectrum disorder and typically developing controls: A systematic review and meta-analysis. *Journal of Autism and Developmental Disorders, 49*(1), 34–43.

CHAPTER 3: WHAT CAUSES AUTISM?

Andalib, S., Emamhadi, M. R., Yousefzadeh-Chabok, S., Shakouri, S. K., Høilund-Carlsen, P. F., Vafaee, M. S., et al. (2017). Maternal SSRI exposure increases the risk of autistic offspring: A meta-analysis and systematic review. *European Psychiatry, 45,* 161–166.

Bernier, R., Golzio, C., Xiong, B., Stessman, H., Coe, B., Penn, O., et al. (2014). Disruptive CHD8 mutations define a subtype of autism early in development. *Cell, 158,* 263–276.

Bernier, R., Hudac, C., Chen, Q., Zeng, C., Wallace, A., Gerdts, J., et al. (2017). Developmental trajectories for young children with 16p11.2 copy number variation. *American Journal of Medical Genetics, Part B: Neuropsychiatric Genetics, 174*(4), 367–380.

Christensen, J., Grønborg, T. K., Sørensen, M. J., Schendel, D., Parner, E. T., Pedersen, L. H., et al. (2013). Prenatal valproate exposure and risk of autism spectrum disorders and childhood autism. *JAMA, 309*(16), 1696–1703.

Coe, B., Stessman, H., Sulovari, A., Geisheker, M., Bakken, T., Lake, A., et al. (2019). Neurodevelopmental disease genes implicated by de novo mutation and CNV morbidity. *Nature Genetics, 51*(1), 106–116.

Conde-Agudelo, A., Rosas-Bermudez, A., & Norton, M. H. (2016). Birth spacing and risk of autism and other neurodevelopmental disabilities: A systematic review. *Pediatrics, 137*(5).

Curran, E. A., O'Neill, S. M., Cryan, J. F., Kenny, L. C., Dinan, T. G., Khashan, A. S., et al. (2015). Research review: Birth by caesarean section and development of autism spectrum disorder and attention-deficit/hyperactivity disorder: A systematic review and meta-analysis. *Journal of Child Psychology and Psychiatry, 56*(5), 500–508.

Geisheker, M., Heymann, G., Wang, T., Coe, B., Turner, T., Stessman, H., et al. (2017). Hotspots of missense mutation identify novel neurodevelopmental disorder genes and functional domains. *Nature Neuroscience, 20*(8), 1043–1051.

Geschwind, D. H. (2011). Genetics of autism spectrum disorders. *Trends in Cognitive Sciences, 15*(9), 409–416.

Green Snyder, L., D'Angelo, D., Chen, Q., Bernier, R., Goin-Kochel, R. P., Wallace, A. S., et al. (2016). Autism spectrum disorder, developmental and psychiatric features in 16p11.2 duplication. *Journal of Autism and Developmental Disorders, 46*(8), 2734–2748.

Guinchat, V., Thorsen, P., Laurent, C., Cans, C., Bodeau, N., & Cohen, D. (2012). Pre-, peri- and neonatal risk factors for autism. *Acta Obstetricia et Gynecologica Scandinavica, 91*(3), 287–300.

Hanson, E., Bernier, R., Porche, K., Jackson, F., Goin-Kochel, R., Green-Snyder, L., et al. (2014). The cognitive and behavioral phenotype of the 16p11.2 deletion in a clinically ascertained population. *Biological Psychiatry, 77*(9), 785–793.

Jiang, H. Y., Xu, L. L., Shao, L., Xia, R. M., Yu, Z. H., Ling, Z. X., et al. (2016). Maternal infection during pregnancy and risk of autism spectrum disorders: A systematic review and meta-analysis. *Brain, Behavior, and Immunity, 58,* 165–172.

Krumm, N., O'Roak, B., Karakoc, E., Mohajeri, K., Nelson, B., Vives, L., et al. (2013). Transmission distortion of small CNVs in sporadic autism. *American Journal of Human Genetics, 93,* 595–606.

Krumm, N., Turner, T., Baker, C., Vives, L., Mohajeri, K., Witherspoon, K., et al. (2015). Excess of rare, inherited truncating mutations in autism. *Nature Genetics, 47*(6), 582–588.

Krupp, D. R., Barnard, R. A., Duffourd, Y., Evans, S. A., Mulqueen, R. M., Bernier, R., et al. (2017). Exonic mosaic mutations contribute risk for autism spectrum disorder. *American Journal of Human Genetics, 101*(3), 369–390.

Lam, J., Sutton, P., Kalkbrenner, A., Windham, G., Halladay, A., Koustas, E., et al. (2016). A systematic review and meta-analysis of multiple airborne pollutants and autism spectrum disorder. *PLOS ONE, 11*(9).

Li, Y. M., Ou, J. J., Liu, L., Zhang, D., Zhao, J. P., & Tang, S. Y. (2016). Association between maternal obesity and autism spectrum disorder in offspring: A meta-analysis. *Journal of Autism and Developmental Disorders, 46*(1), 95–102.

Modabbernia, A., Velthorst, E., & Reichenberg, A. (2017). Environmental risk factors for autism: An evidence-based review of systematic reviews and meta-analyses. *Molecular Autism, 8*(1), 13.

O'Roak, B., Vives, L., Fu, W., Egertson, J., Stanaway, I., Phelps, I., et al. (2012). Massively multiplex targeted sequencing identifies genes recurrently disrupted in autism spectrum disorders. *Science, 338,* 1619–1622.

O'Roak, B., Vives, L., Girirajan, S., Karakoc, E., Krumm, N., Coe, B., et al. (2012).

Sporadic autism exomes reveal a highly interconnected protein network of de novo mutations. *Nature, 485,* 246–250.

Ramaswami, G., & Geschwind, D. H. (2018). Genetics of autism spectrum disorder. *Handbook of Clinical Neurology, 147,* 321–329.

Saghazadeh, A., & Rezaei, N. (2017). Systematic review and meta-analysis links autism and toxic metals and highlights the impact of country development status: Higher blood and erythrocyte levels for mercury and lead, and higher hair antimony, cadmium, lead, and mercury. *Progress in Neuro-Psychopharmacology and Biological Psychiatry, 79,* 340–368.

Sanders, S. J., Campbell, A. J., Cottrell, J. R., Moller, R. S., Wagner, F. F., Auldridge, A. L., et al. (2018). Progress in understanding and treating SCN2A-mediated disorders. *Trends in Neuroscience, 41*(7), 442–456.

Sestan, N., & State, M. W. (2018). Lost in translation: Traversing the complex path from genomics to therapeutics in autism spectrum disorder. *Neuron, 100*(2), 406–423.

Stessman, H., Bernier, R., & Eichler, E. (2014). A genotype-first approach to defining the subtypes of a complex disease. *Cell, 156*(5), 872–877.

Stessman, H., Xiong, B., Coe, B., Wang, T., Hoekzema, K., Fenckova, M., et al. (2017). Targeted sequencing identifies 91 neurodevelopmental disorder risk genes with autism and developmental disability biases. *Nature Genetics, 49*(4), 515–526.

Tebbenkamp, A. T., Willsey, A. J., State, M. W., & Šestan, N. (2014). The developmental transcriptome of the human brain: Implications for neurodevelopmental disorders. *Current Opinion in Neurology, 27*(2), 149.

Thye, M. D., Bednarz, H. M., Herringshaw, A. J., Sartin, E. B., & Kana, R. K. (2018). The impact of atypical sensory processing on social impairments in autism spectrum disorder. *Developmental Cognitive Neuroscience, 29,* 151–167.

Wang, C., Geng, H., Liu, W., & Zhang, G. (2017). Prenatal, perinatal, and postnatal factors associated with autism: A meta-analysis. *Medicine, 96*(18).

Weiner, D. J., Wigdor, E. M., Ripke, S., Walters, R. K., Kosmicki, J. A., Grove, J., et al. (2017). Polygenic transmission disequilibrium confirms that common and rare variation act additively to create risk for autism spectrum disorders. *Nature Genetics, 49*(7), 978–985.

Woodbury-Smith, M., & Scherer, S. W. (2018). Progress in the genetics of autism spectrum disorder. *Developmental Medicine and Child Neurology, 60*(5), 445–451.

Yuen, R. K., Szatmari, P., & Vorstman, J. A. (2019). Genetics of autism spectrum. In F. Volkmar (Ed.), *Autism and pervasive developmental disorders* (pp. 112–128). Cambridge, UK: Cambridge University Press.

Zheng, Z., Zhang, L., Li, S., Zhao, F., Wang, Y., Huang, L., et al. (2017). Association among obesity, overweight and autism spectrum disorder: A systematic review and meta-analysis. *Scientific Reports, 7*(1), 11697.

CHAPTER 4: HOW DOES THE BRAIN DEVELOP DIFFERENTLY IN AUTISM?

Baron-Cohen, S., Ring, H., Bullmore, E., Wheelwright, S., Ashwin, C., & Williams, S. (2000). The amygdala theory of autism. *Neuroscience and Biobehavioral Reviews, 24,* 355–364.

Blakemore, S.-J. (2008). The social brain in adolescence. *Nature Reviews Neuroscience 9*(4), 267.

Dawson, G., Jones, E. J., Merkle, K., Venema, K., Lowy, R., Faja, S., et al. (2012). Early behavioral intervention is associated with normalized brain activity in young children with autism. *Journal of the American Academy of Child Adolescent Psychiatry, 51,* 1550–1559.

Dawson, G., Rogers, S., Munson, J., Smith, M., Winter, J., Greenson, J., et al. (2010). Randomized, controlled trial of an intervention for toddlers with autism: The Early Start Denver Model. *Pediatrics, 125,* 17–23.

Ecker, C., Bookheimer, S. Y., & Murphy, D. G. (2015). Neuroimaging in autism spectrum disorder: Brain structure and function across the lifespan. *The Lancet Neurology, 14*(11), 1121–1134.

Faja, S., Webb, S. J., Jones, E., Merkle, K., Kamara, D., Bavaro, J., et al. (2012). The effects of face expertise training on the behavioral performance and brain activity of adults with high functioning autism spectrum disorders. *Journal of Autism and Developmental Disorders, 42*(2), 278–293.

Ha, S., Sohn, I. J., Kim, N., Sim, H. J., & Cheon, K. A. (2015). Characteristics of brains in autism spectrum disorder: Structure, function and connectivity across the lifespan. *Experimental Neurobiology, 24*(4), 273–284.

Hull, J. V., Jacokes, Z. J., Torgerson, C. M., Irimia, A., & Van Horn, J. D. (2017). Resting-state functional connectivity in autism spectrum disorders: A review. *Frontiers in Psychiatry, 7,* 205.

Kaiser, M. D., Hudac, C. M., Shultz, S., Lee, S. M., Cheung, C., Berken, A. M., et al. (2010). Neural signatures of autism. *Proceedings of the National Academy of Sciences of the USA, 107,* 21223–21228.

Kandel, E., Schwartz, J., Jessell, T., Siegelbaum, S., & Hudspeth, A. (2012). *Principles of neural science* (5th ed.). New York: McGraw-Hill Education.

Konrad, K., Firk, C., & Uhlhaas, P. J. (2013). Brain development during adolescence: Neuroscientific insights into this developmental period. *Deutsches Ärzteblatt International, 110*(25), 425.

Lenroot, R. K., & Giedd, J. N. (2006). Brain development in children and adolescents: Insights from anatomical magnetic resonance imaging. *Neuroscience and Biobehavioral Reviews, 30*(6), 718–729.

Li, D., Karnath, H. O., & Xu, X. (2017). Candidate biomarkers in children with autism spectrum disorder: A review of MRI studies. *Neuroscience Bulletin, 33*(2), 219–237.

McPartland, J., Tillman, R., Yang, D., Bernier, R., & Pelphrey, K. (2014). The social neuroscience of autism spectrum disorder. In F. Volkmar, R. Paul, A. Klin, & D. Cohen (Eds.), *Handbook of autism and pervasive developmental disorders* (4th ed.). New York: Wiley.

Müller, R. A., & Fishman, I. (2018). Brain connectivity and neuroimaging of social networks in autism. *Trends in Cognitive Sciences, 22*(12), 1103–1116.

O'Reilly, C., Lewis, J. D., & Elsabbagh, M. (2017). Is functional brain connectivity atypical in autism?: A systematic review of EEG and MEG studies. *PLOS ONE, 12*(5), e0175870.

Pagnozzi, A. M., Conti, E., Calderoni, S., Fripp, J., & Rose, S. E. (2018). A systematic review of structural MRI biomarkers in autism spectrum disorder: A machine learning perspective. *International Journal of Developmental Neuroscience, 71,* 68–82.

Rane, P., Cochran, D., Hodge, S. M., Haselgrove, C., Kennedy, D., & Frazier, J. A.

(2015). Connectivity in autism: A review of MRI connectivity studies. *Harvard Review of Psychiatry, 23*(4), 223.

Ventola, P., Friedman, H. E., Anderson, L. C., Wolf, J. M., Oosting, D., Foss-Feig, J., et al. (2014). Improvements in social and adaptive functioning following short-duration PRT program: A clinical replication. *Journal of Autism and Developmental Disorders, 44*(11), 2862–2870.

Yang, D., Pelphrey, K. A., Sukhodolsky, D. G., Crowley, M. J., Dayan, E., Dvornek, N. C., et al. (2016). Brain responses to biological motion predict treatment outcome in young children with autism. *Translational Psychiatry, 6*(11), p. e948.

CHAPTER 5: WHAT ARE THE BEST PRACTICES FOR HELPING A CHILD WITH AUTISM?

Adams, K. E., Cohen, M. H., Eisenberg, D., & Jonsen, A. R. (2002). Ethical considerations of complementary and alternative medical therapies in conventional medical settings. *Annals of Internal Medicine, 137*(8), 660–664.

Barroso, N. E., Mendez, L., Graziano, P. A., & Bagner, D. M. (2018). Parenting stress through the lens of different clinical groups: A systematic review and meta-analysis. *Journal of Abnormal Child Psychology, 46*(3), 449–461.

Benvenuto, A., Battan, B., Porfirio, M. C., & Curatolo, P. (2013). Pharmacotherapy of autism spectrum disorders. *Brain and Development, 35*(2), 119–127.

Bernier, R., Stevens, A., & Ankenman, K. (2014). Assessment of core features of ASD. In P. Sturmey, J. Tarbox, D. Dixon, & J. L. Matson (Eds.), *Handbook of early intervention for autism spectrum disorders: Research, practice, and policy.* New York: Springer.

Cowan, R. J., Abel, L., & Candel, L. (2017). A meta-analysis of single-subject research on behavioral momentum to enhance success in students with autism. *Journal of Autism and Developmental Disorders, 47*(5), 1464–1477.

Dawson, G. (2013). Early intensive behavioral intervention appears beneficial for young children with autism spectrum disorders. *Journal of Pediatrics, 162*(5), 1080–1081.

Dawson, G., & Burner, K. (2011). Behavioral interventions in children and adolescents with autism spectrum disorder: A review of recent findings. *Current Opinion in Pediatrics, 23*(6), 616–620.

Dawson, G., Jones, E. J., Merkle, K., Venema, K., Lowy, R., Faja, S., et al. (2012). Early behavioral intervention is associated with normalized brain activity in young children with autism. *Journal of the American Academy of Child and Adolescent Psychiatry, 51,* 1550–1559.

Dawson, G., Rogers, S., Munson, J., Smith, M., Winter, J., Greenson, J., et al. (2010). Randomized, controlled trial of an intervention for toddlers with autism: The Early Start Denver Model. *Pediatrics, 125,* 17–23.

Estes, A., Olson, E., Munson, J., Sullivan, K., Greenson, J., Winter, J., et al. (2013). Parenting-related stress and psychological distress in mothers of toddlers with autism spectrum disorders. *Brain and Development, 35,* 133–138.

Gates, J. A., Kang, E., & Lerner, M. D. (2017). Efficacy of group social skills interventions for youth with autism spectrum disorder: A systematic review and meta-analysis. *Clinical Psychology Review, 52,* 164–181.

Goldstein, S., & Ozonoff, S. (Eds.). (2018). *Assessment of autism spectrum disorder.* New York: Guilford Press.

Gringras, P., Nir, T., Breddy, J., Frydman-Marom, A., & Findling, R. L. (2017). Efficacy and safety of pediatric prolonged-release melatonin for insomnia in children with autism spectrum disorder. *Journal of the American Academy of Child and Adolescent Psychiatry, 56*(11), 948–957.

Gulliver, D., Werry, E., Reekie, T. A., Katte, T. A., Jorgensen, W., & Kassiou, M. (2018). Targeting the oxytocin system: New pharmacotherapeutic approaches. *Trends in Pharmacological Sciences, 40*(1), 22–37.

Howes, O. D., Rogdaki, M., Findon, J. L., Wichers, R. H., Charman, T., King, B. H., et al. (2018). Autism spectrum disorder: Consensus guidelines on assessment, treatment and research from the British Association for Psychopharmacology. *Journal of Psychopharmacology, 32*(1), 3–29.

Keech, B., Crowe, S., & Hocking, D. R. (2018). Intranasal oxytocin, social cognition and neurodevelopmental disorders: A meta-analysis. *Psychoneuroendocrinology, 87,* 9–19.

Koegel, R. L., Koegel, L. K., Kim, S., Bradshaw, J., Gengoux, G. W., Vismara, L. A., et al. (2018). *Pivotal response treatment for autism spectrum disorders.* Baltimore: Brookes.

Lord, C., Rutter, M., DiLavore, P. C., Risi, S., Gotham, K., & Bishop, S. L. (2012). *Autism Diagnostic Observation Schedule (ADOS-2) modules 1–4.* Los Angeles: Western Psychological Services.

Lord, C., Rutter, M., & Le Couteur, A. (1994). Autism Diagnostic Interview—Revised: A revised version of a diagnostic interview for caregivers of individuals with possible pervasive developmental disorders. *Journal of Autism and Developmental Disorders, 24*(5), 659–685.

Masi, A., Lampit, A., DeMayo, M. M., Glozier, N., Hickie, I. B., & Guastella, A. J. (2017). A comprehensive systematic review and meta-analysis of pharmacological and dietary supplement interventions in paediatric autism: Moderators of treatment response and recommendations for future research. *Psychological Medicine, 47*(7), 1323–1334.

McPheeters, M. L., Warren, Z., Sathe, N., Bruzek, J. L., Krishnaswami, S., Jerome, R. N., et al. (2011). A systematic review of medical treatments for children with autism spectrum disorders. *Pediatrics, 127*(5), e1312–e1321.

Myers, S. M., & Johnson, C. P. (2007). Management of children with autism spectrum disorders. *Pediatrics, 120*(5), 1162–1182.

Ozonoff, S., Dawson, G., & McPartland, J. (2014). *A parent's guide to Asperger syndrome and high-functioning autism: How to meet the challenges and help your child thrive* (2nd ed.). New York: Guilford Press.

Peters-Scheffer, N., Didden, R., Korzilius, H., & Sturmey, P. (2011). A meta-analytic study on the effectiveness of comprehensive ABA-based early intervention programs for children with autism spectrum disorders. *Research in Autism Spectrum Disorders, 5*(1), 60–69.

Postorino, V., Sharp, W. G., McCracken, C. E., Bearss, K., Burrell, T. L., Evans, A. N., et al. (2017). A systematic review and meta-analysis of parent training for disruptive behavior in children with autism spectrum disorder. *Clinical Child and Family Psychology Review, 20*(4), 391–402.

Reichow, B. (2012). Overview of meta-analyses on early intensive behavioral intervention for young children with autism spectrum disorders. *Journal of Autism and Developmental Disorders, 42*(4), 512–520.

Reichow, B., Barton, E. E., Boyd, B. A., & Hume, K. (2012). Early intensive behavioral intervention (EIBI) for young children with autism spectrum disorders (ASD). *Cochrane Database of Systematic Reviews, 10.*

Rogers, S. J., & Dawson, G. (2010). *Early Start Denver Model curriculum checklist for young children with autism.* New York: Guilford Press.

Rogers, S. J., & Dawson, G. (2010). *Early Start Denver Model for young children with autism: Promoting language, learning, and engagement.* New York: Guilford Press.

Rogers, S. J., Dawson, G., & Vismara, L. (2012). *An early start for your child with autism.* New York: Guilford Press.

Schopler, E., Reichler, R. J., DeVellis, R. F., & Daly, K. (1980). Toward objective classification of childhood autism: Childhood Autism Rating Scale (CARS). *Journal of Autism and Developmental Disorders, 10*(1), 91–103.

Sipes, M., & Matson, J. (2014). Measures used to screen and diagnose ASD in young children. In P. Sturmey, J. Tarbox, D. Dixon, & J. L. Matson (Eds.), *Handbook of early intervention for autism spectrum disorders: Research, practice, and policy.* New York: Springer.

South, M., Williams, B. J., McMahon, W. M., Owley, T., Filipek, P. A., Shernoff, E., et al. (2002). Utility of the Gilliam Autism Rating Scale in research and clinical populations. *Journal of Autism and Developmental Disorders, 32*(6), 593–599.

Tachibana, Y., Miyazaki, C., Ota, E., Mori, R., Hwang, Y., Kobayashi, E., et al. (2017). A systematic review and meta-analysis of comprehensive interventions for pre-school children with autism spectrum disorder (ASD). *PLOS ONE, 12*(12), e0186502.

U.S. Department of Education. *Individuals with Disabilities Education Act.* Retrieved from *https://sites.ed.gov/idea.*

Vivanti, G., Duncan, E., Dawson, G., & Rogers, S. J. (2016). *Implementing the group-based Early Start Denver Model for preschoolers with autism.* New York: Springer.

Wagner, S., & Harony-Nicolas, H. (2018). Oxytocin and animal models for autism spectrum disorder. *Current Topics in Behavioral Neuroscience, 35,* 213–237.

Warren, Z., McPheeters, M. L., Sathe, N., Foss-Feig, J. H., Glasser, A., & Veenstra-VanderWeele, J. (2011). A systematic review of early intensive intervention for autism spectrum disorders. *Pediatrics, 127*(5), e1303–e1311.

Weston, L., Hodgkins, J., & Langdon, P. E. (2016). Effectiveness of cognitive behavioural therapy with people who have autistic spectrum disorders: A systematic review and meta-analysis. *Clinical Psychology Review, 49,* 41–54.

Yamasue, H., & Domes, G. (2018). Oxytocin and autism spectrum disorders. *Current Topics in Behavioral Neuroscience, 35,* 449–465.

Zwaigenbaum, L., & Penner, M. (2018). Autism spectrum disorder: Advances in diagnosis and evaluation. *BMJ, 361,* k1674.

CHAPTER 6: EXERCISE, SLEEP, AND ASD

American Academy of Pediatrics. (2016). Recommended amount of sleep for pediatric populations. *Pediatrics, 138*(2), e20161601.

Archer, T., & Kostrzewa, R. M. (2015). Physical exercise alleviates health defects, symptoms, and biomarkers in schizophrenia spectrum disorder. *Neurotoxicity Research, 28*(3), 268–280.

Auger, R. R., Burgess, H. J., Emens, J. S., Deriy, L. V., Thomas, S. M., & Sharkey, K. M.

(2015). Clinical practice guideline for the treatment of intrinsic circadian rhythm sleep-wake disorders: Advanced sleep-wake phase disorder (ASWPD), delayed sleep-wake phase disorder (DSWPD), non-24-hour sleep-wake rhythm disorder (N24SWD), and irregular sleep-wake rhythm disorder (ISWRD). *Journal of Clinical Sleep Medicine, 11*(10), 1199–1236.

Bandini, L. G., Gleason, J., Curtin, C., Lividini, K., Anderson, S. E., Cermak, S. A., et al. (2013). Comparison of physical activity between children with autism spectrum disorders and typically developing children. *Autism, 17*(1), 44–54.

Barnes, C. M., & Drake, C. L. (2015). Prioritizing sleep health: Public health policy recommendations. *Perspectives on Psychological Science, 10*(6), 733–737.

Bremer, E., Crozier, M., & Lloyd, M. (2016). A systematic review of the behavioural outcomes following exercise interventions for children and youth with autism spectrum disorder. *Autism, 20*(8), 899–915.

Bruni, O., Alonso-Alconada, D., Besag, F., Biran, V., Braam, W., Cortese, S., et al. (2015). Current role of melatonin in pediatric neurology: Clinical recommendations. *European Journal of Paediatric Neurology, 19*(2), 122–133.

Burdette, H. L., & Whitaker, R. C. (2005). Resurrecting free play in young children: Looking beyond fitness and fatness to attention, affiliation, and affect. *Archives of Pediatric and Adolescent Medicine, 159*(1), 46–50.

Chang, A. M., Aeschbach, D., Duffy, J. F., & Czeisler, C. A. (2015). Evening use of light-emitting eReaders negatively affects sleep, circadian timing, and next-morning alertness. *Proceedings of the National Academy of Sciences of the USA, 112,* 1232–1237.

Cuomo, B. M., Vaz, S., Lee, E. A. L., Thompson, C., Rogerson, J. M., & Falkmer, T. (2017). Effectiveness of sleep-based interventions for children with autism spectrum disorder: A meta synthesis. *Pharmacotherapy, 37*(5), 555–578.

De Paz, A. M., Sanchez-Mut, J. V., Samitier-Martí, M., Petazzi, P., Sáez, M., Szczesna, K., et al. (2015). Circadian cycle-dependent MeCP2 and brain chromatin changes. *PLOS ONE, 10*(4), e0123693.

Denham, J., Marques, F. Z., O'Brien, B. J., & Charchar, F. J. (2014). Exercise: Putting action into our epigenome. *Sports Medicine, 44*(2), 189–209.

Devnani, P. A., & Hegde, A. U. (2015). Autism and sleep disorders. *Journal of Pediatric Neurosciences, 10*(4), 304.

Dillon, S. R., Adams, D., Goudy, L., Bittner, M., & McNamara, S. (2017). Evaluating exercise as evidence-based practice for individuals with autism spectrum disorder. *Frontiers in Public Health, 4,* 290.

Falbe, J., Davison, K. K., Franckle, R. L., Ganter, C., Gortmaker, S. L., Smith, L., et al. (2015). Sleep duration, restfulness, and screens in the sleep environment. *Pediatrics, 135*(2), e367–e375.

Goldman, S. E., Alder, M. L., Burgess, H. J., Corbett, B. A., Hundley, R., Wofford, D., et al. (2017). Characterizing sleep in adolescents and adults with autism spectrum disorders. *Journal of Autism and Developmental Disorders, 47*(6), 1682–1695.

Gómez, R. L., & Edgin, J. O. (2015). Sleep as a window into early neural development: Shifts in sleep-dependent learning effects across early childhood. *Child Development Perspectives, 9*(3), 183–189.

Hackney, A. C. (2015). Epigenetic aspects of exercise on stress reactivity. *Psychoneuroendocrinology, 61,* 17.

Hargreaves, M. (2015). Exercise and gene expression. *Progress in Molecular Biology and Translational Science, 135,* 457–469.

Healy, S., Nacario, A., Braithwaite, R. E., & Hopper, C. (2018). The effect of physical activity interventions on youth with autism spectrum disorder: A meta-analysis. *Autism Research, 11*(6), 818–833.

Hillman, C. H. (2014). The relation of childhood physical activity and aerobic fitness to brain function and cognition: A review. *Monographs of the Society for Research in Child Development, 79,* 1–6.

Horváth, K., Myers, K., Foster, R., & Plunkett, K. J. (2015). Napping facilitates word learning in early lexical development. *Sleep Research, 24*(5), 503–509.

Jones, R. A., Downing, K., Rinehart, N. J., Barnett, L. M., May, T., McGillivray, J. A., et al. (2017). Physical activity, sedentary behavior and their correlates in children with autism spectrum disorder: A systematic review. *PLOS ONE, 12*(2), e0172482.

Kashimoto, R. K., Toffoli, L. V., Manfredo, M. H., Volpini, V. L., Martins-Pinge, M. C., Pelosi, G., et al. (2016). Physical exercise affects the epigenetic programming of rat brain and modulates the adaptive response evoked by repeated restraint stress. *Behavioural Brain Research, 296,* 286–289.

Khan, N. A., & Hillman, C. H. (2014). Benefits of regular aerobic exercise for executive functioning in healthy populations. *Pediatric Exercise Science, 26,* 138–146.

Maski, K. P. (2015). Sleep-dependent memory consolidation in children. *Seminars in Pediatric Neurology, 22*(2), 130–134.

Must, A., Phillips, S. M., Curtin, C., Anderson, S. E., Maslin, M., Lividini, K., et al. (2014). Comparison of sedentary behaviors between children with autism spectrum disorders and typically developing children. *Autism, 18*(4), 376–384.

Myer, G. D., Faigenbaum, A. D., Edwards, N. M., Clark, J. F., Best, T. M., & Sallis, R. E. (2015). Sixty minutes of what?: A developing brain perspective for activating children with an integrative exercise approach. *British Journal of Sports Medicine, 49*(23), 1510–1516.

Reynolds, A. M., & Malow, B. A. (2011). Sleep and autism spectrum disorders. *Pediatric Clinics, 58*(3), 685–698.

Richdale, A. L., & Schreck, K. A. (2009). Sleep problems in autism spectrum disorders: Prevalence, nature, and possible biopsychosocial aetiologies. *Sleep Medicine Reviews, 13*(6), 403–411.

Rodrigues, G. M., Jr., Toffoli, L. V., Manfredo, M. H., Francis-Oliveira, J., Silva, A. S., Raquel, H. A., et al. (2015). Acute stress affects the global DNA methylation profile in rat brain: Modulation by physical exercise. *Behavioural Brain Research, 15*(279), 123–128.

Schuch, J. B., Genro, J. P., Bastos, C. R., Ghisleni, G., & Tovo-Rodrigues, L. (2018). The role of CLOCK gene in psychiatric disorders: Evidence from human and animal research. *American Journal of Medical Genetics Part B: Neuropsychiatric Genetics, 177*(2), 181–198.

Singh, A., Uijtdewilligen, L., Twisk, J. W., van Mechelen, W., & Chinapaw, M. J. (2012). Physical activity and performance at school: A systematic review of the literature including a methodological quality assessment. *Archives of Pediatric and Adolescent Medicine, 166*(1), 49–55.

Souders, M. C., Zavodny, S., Eriksen, W., Sinko, R., Connell, J., Kerns, C., et al. (2017).

Sleep in children with autism spectrum disorder. *Current Psychiatry Reports, 19*(6), 34.

Tan, B. W., Pooley, J. A., & Speelman, C. P. (2016). A meta-analytic review of the efficacy of physical exercise interventions on cognition in individuals with autism spectrum disorder and ADHD. *Journal of Autism and Developmental Disorders, 46*(9), 3126–3143.

Urbain, C., De Tiège, X., Op De Beeck, M., Bourguignon, M., Wens, V., Verheulpen D., et al. (2016). Sleep in children triggers rapid reorganization of memory-related brain processes. *NeuroImage, 134*, 213–222.

von Schantz, M., & Archer, S. N. (2003). Clocks, genes and sleep. *Journal of the Royal Society of Medicine, 96*(10), 486–489.

CHAPTER 7: GASTROINTESTINAL AND FEEDING PROBLEMS, FOOD, AND DIET IN ASD

Bubnov, R. V., Spivak, M. Y., Lazarenko, L. M., Bomba, A., & Boyko, N. V. (2015). Probiotics and immunity: Provisional role for personalized diets and disease prevention. *EPMA Journal, 6*(1), 14.

Buie, T., Campbell, D. B., Fuchs, G. J., Furuta, G. T., Levy, J., VandeWater, J., et al. (2010). Evaluation, diagnosis, and treatment of gastrointestinal disorders in individuals with ASDs: A consensus report. *Pediatrics, 125*(Suppl. 1), S1–S18.

Cao, X., Lin, P., Jiang, P., & Li, C. (2013). Characteristics of the gastrointestinal microbiome in children with autism spectrum disorder: A systematic review. *Shanghai Archives of Psychiatry, 25*(6), 342.

Castro, K., Faccioli, L. S., Baronio, D., Gottfried, C., Perry, I. S., & Riesgo, R. D. S. (2015). Effect of a ketogenic diet on autism spectrum disorder: A systematic review. *Research in Autism Spectrum Disorders, 20*, 31–38.

Castro, K., Klein, L. D. S., Baronio, D., Gottfried, C., Riesgo, R., & Perry, I. S. (2016). Folic acid and autism: What do we know? *Nutritional Neuroscience, 19*(7), 310–317.

Chistol, L. T., Bandini, L. G., Must, A., Phillips, S., Cermak, S. A., & Curtin, C. (2018). Sensory sensitivity and food selectivity in children with autism spectrum disorder. *Journal of Autism and Developmental Disorders, 48*(2), 583–591.

Esteban-Figuerola, P., Canals, J., Fernández-Cao, J. C., & Arija Val, V. (2018). Differences in food consumption and nutritional intake between children with autism spectrum disorders and typically developing children: A meta-analysis. *Autism, 23*(5), 1079–1095. [Epub ahead of print]

Fulceri, F., Morelli, M., Santocchi, E., Cena, H., Del Bianco, T., Narzisi, A., et al. (2016). Gastrointestinal symptoms and behavioral problems in preschoolers with autism spectrum disorder. *Digestive and Liver Disease, 48*(3), 248–254.

Gogou, M., & Kolios, G. (2017). The effect of dietary supplements on clinical aspects of autism spectrum disorder: A systematic review of the literature. *Brain and Development, 39*(8), 656–664.

Gorrindo, P., Williams, K. C., Lee, E. B., Walker, L. S., McGrew, S. G., & Levitt, P. (2012). Gastrointestinal dysfunction in autism: Parental report, clinical evaluation, and associated factors. *Autism Research, 5*(2), 101–108.

Grayson, D. S., Kroenke, C. D., Neuringer, M., & Fair, D. A. (2014). Dietary omega-3 fatty acids modulate large-scale systems organization in the rhesus macaque brain. *Journal of Neuroscience, 34*(6), 2065–2074.

Holingue, C., Newill, C., Lee, L. C., Pasricha, P. J., & Daniele Fallin, M. (2018). Gastrointestinal symptoms in autism spectrum disorder: A review of the literature on ascertainment and prevalence. *Autism Research, 11*(1), 24–36.

Israelyan, N., & Margolis, K. G. (2018). Serotonin as a link between the gut-brain-microbiome axis in autism spectrum disorders. *Pharmacological Research, 132,* 1–6.

Kang, V., Wagner, G. C., & Ming, X. (2014). Gastrointestinal dysfunction in children with autism spectrum disorders. *Autism Research, 7*(4), 501–506.

Kopec, A. M., Fiorentino, M. R., & Bilbo, S. D. (2018). Gut-immune-brain dysfunction in autism: Importance of sex. *Brain Research, 1693*(Part B), 214–217.

Lange, K. W., Hauser, J., & Reissmann, A. (2015). Gluten-free and casein-free diets in the therapy of autism. *Current Opinion in Clinical Nutrition and Metabolic Care, 18*(6), 572–575.

Levine, S. Z., Kodesh, A., Viktorin, A., Smith, L., Uher, R., Reichenberg, A., et al. (2018). Association of maternal use of folic acid and multivitamin supplements in the periods before and during pregnancy with the risk of autism spectrum disorder in offspring. *JAMA Psychiatry, 75*(2), 176–184.

Li, Q., Han, Y., Dy, A. B. C., & Hagerman, R. J. (2017). The gut microbiota and autism spectrum disorders. *Frontiers in Cellular Neuroscience, 11,* 120.

Li, Y. J., Ou, J. J., Li, Y. M., & Xiang, D. X. (2017). Dietary supplement for core symptoms of autism spectrum disorder: Where are we now and where should we go? *Frontiers in Psychiatry, 8,* 155.

Ly, V., Bottelier, M., Hoekstra, P. J., Vasquez, A. A., Buitelaar, J. K., & Rommelse, N. N. (2017). Elimination diets' efficacy and mechanisms in attention deficit hyperactivity disorder and autism spectrum disorder. *European Child and Adolescent Psychiatry, 26*(9), 1067–1079.

Maqsood, R., & Stone, T. W. (2016). The gut-brain axis, BDNF, NMDA and CNS disorders. *Neurochemical Resesarch, 11,* 2819–2835.

Masi, A., Lampit, A., DeMayo, M. M., Glozier, N., Hickie, I. B., & Guastella, A. J. (2017). A comprehensive systematic review and meta-analysis of pharmacological and dietary supplement interventions in paediatric autism: Moderators of treatment response and recommendations for future research. *Psychological Medicine, 47*(7), 1323–1334.

Mayer, E. A., Tillisch, K., & Gupta, A. (2015). Gut/brain axis and the microbiota. *Journal of Clinical Investigation, 125*(3), 926–938.

McCue, L. M., Flick, L. H., Twyman, K. A., & Xian, H. (2017). Gastrointestinal dysfunctions as a risk factor for sleep disorders in children with idiopathic autism spectrum disorder: A retrospective cohort study. *Autism, 21*(8), 1010–1020.

McElhanon, B. O., McCracken, C., Karpen, S., & Sharp, W. G. (2014). Gastrointestinal symptoms in autism spectrum disorder: A meta-analysis. *Pediatrics, 133*(5), 872–883.

Mittal, R., Debs, L. H., Patel, A. P., Nguyen, D., Patel, K., O'Connor, G., et al. (2016). Neurotransmitters: The critical modulators regulating gut-brain axis. *Journal of Cell Physiology, 232*(9), 2359–2372.

Moody, L., Chen, H., & Pan, Y. X. (2017). Early-life nutritional programming of cognition—the fundamental role of epigenetic mechanisms in mediating the relation between early-life environment and learning and memory process. *Advances in Nutrition, 8*(2), 337–350.

Neuhaus, E., Bernier, R. A., Tham, S. W., & Webb, S. J. (2018). Gastrointestinal and psychiatric symptoms among children and adolescents with autism spectrum disorder. *Frontiers in Psychiatry, 9*(515), 1–9.

Pennesi, C. M., & Klein, L. C. (2012). Effectiveness of the gluten-free, casein-free diet for children diagnosed with autism spectrum disorder: Based on parental report. *Nutritional Neuroscience, 15*(2), 85–91.

Petra, A. I., Panagiotidou, S., Hatziagelaki, E., Stewart, J. M., Conti, P., & Theoharides, T. C. (2015). Gut-microbiota-brain axis and its effect on neuropsychiatric disorders with suspected immune dysregulation. *Clinical Therapeutics, 37*(5), 984–995.

Piwowarczyk, A., Horvath, A., Łukasik, J., Pisula, E., & Szajewska, H. (2017). Gluten- and casein-free diet and autism spectrum disorders in children: A systematic review. *European Journal of Nutrition, 57*(2), 433–440.

Sable, P., Randhir, K., Kale, A., Chavan-Gautam, P., & Joshi, S. (2015). Maternal micronutrients and brain global methylation patterns in the offspring. *Nutritional Neuroscience, 18*(1), 30–36.

Sathe, N., Andrews, J. C., McPheeters, M. L., & Warren, Z. E. (2017). Nutritional and dietary interventions for autism spectrum disorder: A systematic review. *Pediatrics, 139*(6), e20170346.

Sharp, W. G., Postorino, V., McCracken, C. E., Berry, R. C., Criado, K. K., Burrell, T. L., et al. (2018). Dietary intake, nutrient status, and growth parameters in children with autism spectrum disorder and severe food selectivity: An electronic medical record review. *Journal of the Academy of Nutrition and Dietetics, 118*(10), 1943–1950.

Sharp, W. G., Volkert, V. M., Scahill, L., McCracken, C. E., & McElhanon, B. (2017). A systematic review and meta-analysis of intensive multidisciplinary intervention for pediatric feeding disorders: How standard is the standard of care? *Journal of Pediatrics, 181,* 116–124.

Strøm, M., Granström, C., Lyall, K., Ascherio, A., & Olsen, S. F. (2018). Folic acid supplementation and intake of folate in pregnancy in relation to offspring risk of autism spectrum disorder. *Psychological Medicine, 48*(6), 1048–1054.

Sullivan, E. L., Nousen, E. K., & Chamlou, K. A. (2014). Maternal high fat diet consumption during the perinatal period programs offspring behavior. *Physiology and Behavior, 123,* 236–242.

Surén, P., Roth, C., Bresnahan, M., Haugen, M., Hornig, M., Hirtz, D., et al. (2013). Association between maternal use of folic acid supplements and risk of autism spectrum disorders in children. *JAMA, 309*(6), 570–577.

Thulasi, V., Steer, R. A., Monteiro, I. M., & Ming, X. (2019). Overall severities of gastrointestinal symptoms in pediatric outpatients with and without autism spectrum disorder. *Autism, 23*(2), 524–530.

Wasilewska, J., & Klukowski, M. (2015). Gastrointestinal symptoms and autism spectrum disorder: Links and risks—a possible new overlap syndrome. *Pediatric Health, Medicine and Therapeutics, 6,* 153.

Wolraich, M. L., Wilson, D. B., & White, J. W. (1995). The effect of sugar on behavior or cognition in children: A meta-analysis. *Journal of the American Medical Association, 274*(20), 1617–1621.

Yang, X. L., Liang, S., Zou, M. Y., Sun, C. H., Han, P. P., Jiang, X. T., et al. (2018). Are gastrointestinal and sleep problems associated with behavioral symptoms of autism spectrum disorder? *Psychiatry Research, 259,* 229–235.

Yarandi, S. S., Peterson, D. A., Treisman, G. J., Moran, T. H., & Pasricha, P. J. (2016). Modulatory effects of gut microbiota on the central nervous system: How gut could play a role in neuropsychiatric health and diseases. *Journal of Neurogastroenterology and Motility, 22*(2), 201–212.

CHAPTER 8: TECHNOLOGY AND ASD: LATEST FINDINGS ON THE PERIL AND THE PROMISE

American Academy of Pediatrics. (2016). Family Media Use Plan. Retrieved from *www.healthychildren.org/English/media/Pages/default.aspx.*

Anderson, C. A., Berkowitz, L., Donnerstein, E., Huesmann, L. R., Johnson, J. D., Linz, D., et al. (2003). The influence of media violence on youth. *Psychological Science in the Public Interest, 4*(3), 81–110.

Bellini, S., & Akullian, J. (2007). A meta-analysis of video modeling and video self-modeling interventions for children and adolescents with autism spectrum disorders. *Exceptional Children, 73*(3), 264–287.

Bushman, B. J. (2016). Violent media and hostile appraisals: A meta-analytic review. *Aggressive Behavior, 42,* 605–613.

Bushman, B. J., & Anderson, C. A. (2001). Media violence and the American public: Scientific facts versus media misinformation. *American Psychologist, 56,* 477–489.

Chonchaiya, W., Nuntnarumit, P., & Pruksananonda, C. (2011). Comparison of television viewing between children with autism spectrum disorder and controls. *Acta Paediatrica, 100*(7), 1033–1037.

Christakis, D. A., Garrison, M. M., Herrenkohl, T., Haggerty, K., Rivara, F. P., Zhou, C., et al. (2013). Modifying media content for preschool children: A randomized controlled trial. *Pediatrics, 131*(3), 431–438.

Christakis, D. A., Gilkerson, J., Richards, J. A., Zimmerman, F. J., Garrison, M. M., Xu, D., et al. (2009). Audible television and decreased adult words, infant vocalizations, and conversational turns: A population-based study. *Archives of Pediatrics and Adolescent Medicine, 163*(6), 554–558.

Christakis, D. A., & Zimmerman, F. J. (2007). Violent television viewing during preschool is associated with antisocial behavior during school age. *Pediatrics, 120*(5), 993–999.

Duch, H., Fisher, E. M., Ensari, I., & Harrington, A. (2013). Screen time use in children under 3 years old: A systematic review of correlates. *International Journal of Behavioral Nutrition and Physical Activity, 10*(1), 102.

Fletcher-Watson, S. (2014). A targeted review of computer-assisted learning for people with autism spectrum disorder: Towards a consistent methodology. Review. *Journal of Autism and Developmental Disorders, 1*(2), 87–100.

Garon, N., Zwaigenbaum, L., Bryson, S., Smith, I. M., Brian, J., Roncadin, C., et al. (2016). Temperament and its association with autism symptoms in a high-risk population. *Journal of Abnormal Child Psychology, 44*(4), 757–769.

Garrison, M. M., & Christakis, D. A. (2012). The impact of a healthy media use intervention on sleep in preschool children. *Pediatrics, 130*(3).

Grynszpan, O., Weiss, P. L., Perez-Diaz, F., & Gal, E. (2014). Innovative technology-based interventions for autism spectrum disorders: A meta-analysis. *Autism, 18*(4), 346–361.

Gwynette, M. F., Sidhu, S. S., & Ceranoglu, T. A. (2018). Electronic screen media use in youth with autism Spectrum disorder. *Child and Adolescent Psychiatric Clinics of North America, 27*(2), 203–219.

Hong, E. R., Ganz, J. B., Mason, R., Morin, K., Davis, J. L., Ninci, J., et al. (2016). The effects of video modeling in teaching functional living skills to persons with ASD: A meta-analysis of single-case studies. *Research in Developmental Disabilities, 57*, 158–169.

Kabali, H. K., Irigoyen, M. M., Nunez-Davis, R., Budacki, J. G., Mohanty, S. H., Leister, K. P., et al. (2015). Exposure and use of mobile media devices by young children. *Pediatrics, 136*(6).

Knight, V., McKissick, B. R., & Saunders, A. (2013). A review of technology-based interventions to teach academic skills to students with autism spectrum disorder. *Journal of Autism and Developmental Disorders, 43*(11), 2628–2648.

Kuo, M. H., Orsmond, G. I., Coster, W. J., & Cohn, E. S. (2014). Media use among adolescents with autism spectrum disorder. *Autism, 18*(8), 914–923.

Lee, C. S., Lam, S. H., Tsang, S. T., Yuen, C. M., & Ng, C. K. (2018). The effectiveness of technology-based intervention in improving emotion recognition through facial expression in people with autism spectrum disorder: A systematic review. *Journal of Autism and Developmental Disorders, 5*(2), 91–104.

Li, K., Jurkowski, J. M., & Davison, K. K. (2013). Social support may buffer the effect of intrafamilial stressors on preschool children's television viewing time in low-income families. *Childhood Obesity, 9*(6), 484–491.

Livingstone, S., & Smith, P. K. (2014). Annual research review: Harms experienced by child users of online and mobile technologies: The nature, prevalence and management of sexual and aggressive risks in the digital age. *Journal of Child Psychology and Psychiatry and Allied Disciplines, 55*(6), 635–654.

Logan, K., Iacono, T., & Trembath, D. (2017). A systematic review of research into aided AAC to increase social-communication functions in children with autism spectrum disorder. *Augmentative and Alternative Communication, 33*(1), 51–64.

Mason, R. A., Ganz, J. B., Parker, R. I., Burke, M. D., & Camargo, S. P. (2012). Moderating factors of video-modeling with other as model: A meta-analysis of single-case studies. *Research in Developmental Disabilities, 33*(4), 1076–1086.

Mazurek, M. O., Shattuck, P. T., Wagner, M., & Cooper, B. P. (2012). Prevalence and correlates of screen-based media use among youths with autism spectrum disorders. *Journal of Autism and Developmental Disorders, 42*(8), 1757–1767.

Mazurek, M. O., & Wenstrup, C. (2013). Television, video game and social media use among children with ASD and typically developing siblings. *Journal of Autism and Developmental Disorders, 43*(6), 1258–1271.

Mesa-Gresa, P., Gil-Gómez, H., Lozano-Quilis, J. A., & Gil-Gómez, J. A. (2018). Effectiveness of virtual reality for children and adolescents with autism spectrum disorder: An evidence-based systematic review. *Sensors, 18*(8), 2486.

Mineo, B. A., Ziegler, W., Gill, S., & Salkin, D. (2009). Engagement with electronic screen media among students with autism spectrum disorders. *Journal of Autism and Developmental Disorders, 39*(1), 172–187.

Montes, G. (2016). Children with autism spectrum disorder and screen time: Results from a large, nationally representative US study. *Academic Pediatrics, 16*(2), 122–128.

Morin, K. L., Ganz, J. B., Gregori, E. V., Foster, M. J., Gerow, S. L., Genç-Tosun, D., et al. (2018). A systematic quality review of high-tech AAC interventions as an evidence-based practice. *Augmentative and Alternative Communication, 34*(2), 104–117.

Nally, B., Houlton, B., & Ralph, S. (2000). Researches in brief: The management of television and video by parents of children with autism. *Autism, 4*(3), 331–337.

Pennisi, P., Tonacci, A., Tartarisco, G., Billeci, L., Ruta, L., Gangemi, S., et al. (2016). Autism and social robotics: A systematic review. *Autism Research, 9*(2), 165–183.

Radesky, J. S., Silverstein, M., Zuckerman, B., & Christakis, D. A. (2014). Infant self-regulation and early childhood media exposure. *Pediatrics, 133*(5), e1172–e1178.

Shane, H. C., & Albert, P. D. (2008). Electronic screen media for persons with autism spectrum disorders: Results of a survey. *Journal of Autism and Developmental Disorders, 38*(8), 1499–1508.

Shane, H. C., Laubscher, E. H., Schlosser, R. W., Flynn, S., Sorce, J. F., & Abramson, J. (2012). Applying technology to visually support language and communication in individuals with autism spectrum disorders. *Journal of Autism and Developmental Disorders, 42*(6), 1228–1235.

Takacs, Z. K., Swart, E. K., & Bus, A. G. (2015). Benefits and pitfalls of multimedia and interactive features in technology-enhanced storybooks: A meta-analysis. *Review of Educational Research, 85*(4), 698–739.

CHAPTER 9: ADOLESCENCE AND AUTISM

Anderson, K. A., Sosnowy, C., Kuo, A. A., & Shattuck, P. T. (2018). Transition of individuals with autism to adulthood: A review of qualitative studies. *Pediatrics, 141*(Suppl. 4), S318–S327.

Ballan, M. S., & Freyer, M. B. (2017). Autism spectrum disorder, adolescence, and sexuality education: Suggested interventions for mental health professionals. *Sexuality and Disability, 35*(2), 261–273.

Bennett, A. E., Miller, J. S., Stollon, N., Prasad, R., & Blum, N. J. (2018). Autism spectrum disorder and transition-aged youth. *Current Psychiatry Reports, 20*(11), 103.

Chen, J., Cohn, E. S., & Orsmond, G. I. (2019). Parents' future visions for their autistic transition-age youth: Hopes and expectations. *Autism, 23*(6), 1363–1372. [Epub ahead of print]

Davignon, M. N., Qian, Y., Massolo, M., & Croen, L. A. (2018). Psychiatric and medical conditions in transition-aged individuals with ASD. *Pediatrics, 141*(Suppl. 4), S335–S345.

Gates, J. A., Kang, E., & Lerner, M. D. (2017). Efficacy of group social skills interventions for youth with autism spectrum disorder: A systematic review and meta-analysis. *Clinical Psychology Review, 52,* 164–181.

George, R., & Stokes, M. A. (2018). Gender identity and sexual orientation in autism spectrum disorder. *Autism, 22*(8), 970–982.

George, R., & Stokes, M. A. (2018). Sexual orientation in autism spectrum disorder. *Autism Research, 11*(1), 133–141.

Glidden, D., Bouman, W. P., Jones, B. A., & Arcelus, J. (2016). Gender dysphoria and autism spectrum disorder: A systematic review of the literature. *Sexual Medicine Reviews, 4*(1), 3–14.

Hancock, G. I., Stokes, M. A., & Mesibov, G. B. (2017). Socio-sexual functioning in autism spectrum disorder: A systematic review and meta-analyses of existing literature. *Autism Research, 10*(11), 1823–1833.

Hatfield, M., Ciccarelli, M., Falkmer, T., & Falkmer, M. (2018). Factors related to successful transition planning for adolescents on the autism spectrum. *Journal of Research in Special Educational Needs, 18*(1), 3–14.

Lappé, M., Lau, L., Dudovitz, R. N., Nelson, B. B., Karp, E. A., & Kuo, A. A. (2018). The diagnostic odyssey of autism spectrum disorder. *Pediatrics, 141*(Suppl. 4), S272–S279.

Paradiz, V., Kelso, S., Nelson, A., & Earl, A. (2018). Essential self-advocacy and transition. *Pediatrics, 141*(Suppl. 4), S373–S377.

Pecora, L. A., Mesibov, G. B., & Stokes, M. A. (2016). Sexuality in high-functioning autism: A systematic review and meta-analysis. *Journal of Autism and Developmental Disorders, 46*(11), 3519–3556.

Shattuck, P. T., Lau, L., Anderson, K. A., & Kuo, A. A. (2018). A national research agenda for the transition of youth with autism. *Pediatrics, 141*(Suppl. 4), S355–S361.

Sosnowy, C., Silverman, C., & Shattuck, P. (2018). Parents' and young adults' perspectives on transition outcomes for young adults with autism. *Autism, 22*(1), 29–39.

Strang, J. F., Meagher, H., Kenworthy, L., de Vries, A. L., Menvielle, E., Leibowitz, S., et al. (2018). Initial clinical guidelines for co-occurring autism spectrum disorder and gender dysphoria or incongruence in adolescents. *Journal of Clinical Child and Adolescent Psychology, 47*(1), 105–115.

Turner, D., Briken, P., & Schöttle, D. (2017). Autism-spectrum disorders in adolescence and adulthood: Focus on sexuality. *Current Opinion in Psychiatry, 30*(6), 409–416.

Van Der Miesen, A. I., Hurley, H., & De Vries, A. L. (2016). Gender dysphoria and autism spectrum disorder: A narrative review. *International Review of Psychiatry, 28*(1), 70–80.

Vincent, J. (2019). It's the fear of the unknown: Transition from higher education for young autistic adults. *Autism, 23*(6), 1575–1585. [Epub ahead of print]

Watkins, L., O'Reilly, M., Kuhn, M., Gevarter, C., Lancioni, G. E., Sigafoos, J., et al. (2015). A review of peer-mediated social interaction interventions for students with autism in inclusive settings. *Journal of Autism and Developmental Disorders, 45*(4), 1070–1083.

White, S. W., Simmons, G. L., Gotham, K. O., Conner, C. M., Smith, I. C., Beck, K. B., et al. (2018). Psychosocial treatments targeting anxiety and depression in adolescents and adults on the autism spectrum: Review of the latest research and recommended future directions. *Current Psychiatry Reports, 20*(10), 82.

CHAPTER 10: ADULTHOOD AND AUTISM

Anderson, D., Liang, J., & Lord, C. (2014). Predicting young adult outcome among more and less cognitively able individuals with autism spectrum disorders. *Journal of Child Psychology and Psychiatry, 55*(5), 485–494.

Dijkhuis, R. R., Ziermans, T. B., Van Rijn, S., Staal, W. G., & Swaab, H. (2017).

Self-regulation and quality of life in high-functioning young adults with autism. *Autism, 21*(7), 896–906.

García-Villamisar, D., & Hughes, C. (2007). Supported employment improves cognitive performance in adults with autism. *Journal of Intellectual Disability Research, 51,* 142–150.

Gelbar, N. W., Smith, I., & Reichow, B. (2014). Systematic review of articles describing experience and supports of individuals with autism enrolled in college and university programs. *Journal of Autism and Developmental Disorders, 44*(10), 2593–2601.

Gotham, K., Brunwasser, S., & Lord, C. (2015). Depressive and anxiety symptom trajectories from school age through young adulthood in samples with autism spectrum disorder and developmental delay. *Journal of American Academy of Child and Adolescent Psychiatry, 54*(5), 369–376.

Hollocks, M., Lerh, J. W., Magiati, I., Meiser-Stedman, R., & Brugha, T. (2018). Anxiety and depression in adults with autism spectrum disorder: A systematic review and meta-analysis. *Psychological Medicine, 49*(4), 559–572.

Levy, A., & Perry, A. (2011). Outcomes in adolescents and adults with autism: A review of the literature. *Research in Autism Spectrum Disorders, 5,* 1271–1282.

Magiati, I., Tay, X. W., & Howlin, P. (2014). Cognitive, language, social, and behavioural outcomes in adults with autism spectrum disorders: A systematic review of longitudinal follow-up studies in adulthood. *Clinical Psychology Review, 34,* 73–86.

Moss, P., Mandy, W., & Howlin, P. (2017). Child and adult factors related to quality of life in adults with autism. *Journal of Autism and Developmental Disorders, 47*(6), 1830–1837.

Nicolaidis, C., Kripke, C. C., & Raymaker, D. (2014). Primary care for adults on the autism spectrum. *Medical Clinics, 98*(5), 1169–1191.

Poon, K. K., & Sidhu, D. J. (2017). Adults with autism spectrum disorders: A review of outcomes, social attainment, and interventions. *Current Opinion in Psychiatry, 30*(2), 77–84.

Scott, M., Milbourn, B., Falkmer, M., Black, M., Bölte, S., Halladay, A., et al. (2019). Factors impacting employment for people with autism spectrum disorder: A scoping review. *Autism, 23*(4), 869–901. [Epub ahead of print]]

Taylor, J. L., McPheeters, M. L., Sathe, N. A., Dove, D., Veenstra-VanderWheele, J., & Warren, Z. (2012). A systematic review of vocational interventions for young adults with autism spectrum disorders. *Pediatrics, 130*(3), 531–538.

Taylor, J. L., & Seltzer, M. M. (2011). Employment and post-secondary educational activities for young adults with autism spectrum disorders during the transition to adulthood. *Journal of Autism and Developmental Disorders, 41*(5), 566–574.

van Heijst, B. F., & Geurts, H. M. (2015). Quality of life in autism across the lifespan: A meta-analysis. *Autism, 19*(2), 158–167.

INDEX

About the Authors

Raphael A. Bernier, PhD, is Executive Director of the Seattle Children's Autism Center, Associate Director of the Center on Human Development and Disability, and Professor of Psychiatry and Behavioral Sciences at the University of Washington. He is an active clinician and researcher whose work focuses on how autism develops, how the brain is involved, and ways to improve the quality of life of individuals with autism spectrum disorder and their families.

Geraldine Dawson, PhD, is the William Cleland Professor of Psychiatry and Behavioral Sciences, Director of the Duke Institute for Brain Sciences, and Director of the Duke Center for Autism and Brain Development at Duke University. An internationally recognized autism expert with a focus on early detection, intervention, and brain plasticity in autism, Dr. Dawson is a passionate advocate for families. She is coauthor of *An Early Start for Your Child with Autism* and *A Parent's Guide to Asperger Syndrome and High-Functioning Autism, Second Edition.*

Joel T. Nigg, PhD, is Director of the Division of Psychology and Professor of Psychiatry, Pediatrics, and Behavioral Neuroscience at Oregon Health and Science University. He is a leading researcher on neurodevelopmental conditions in children, as well as a practicing clinician. He is the author of the parent guide *Getting Ahead of ADHD.*